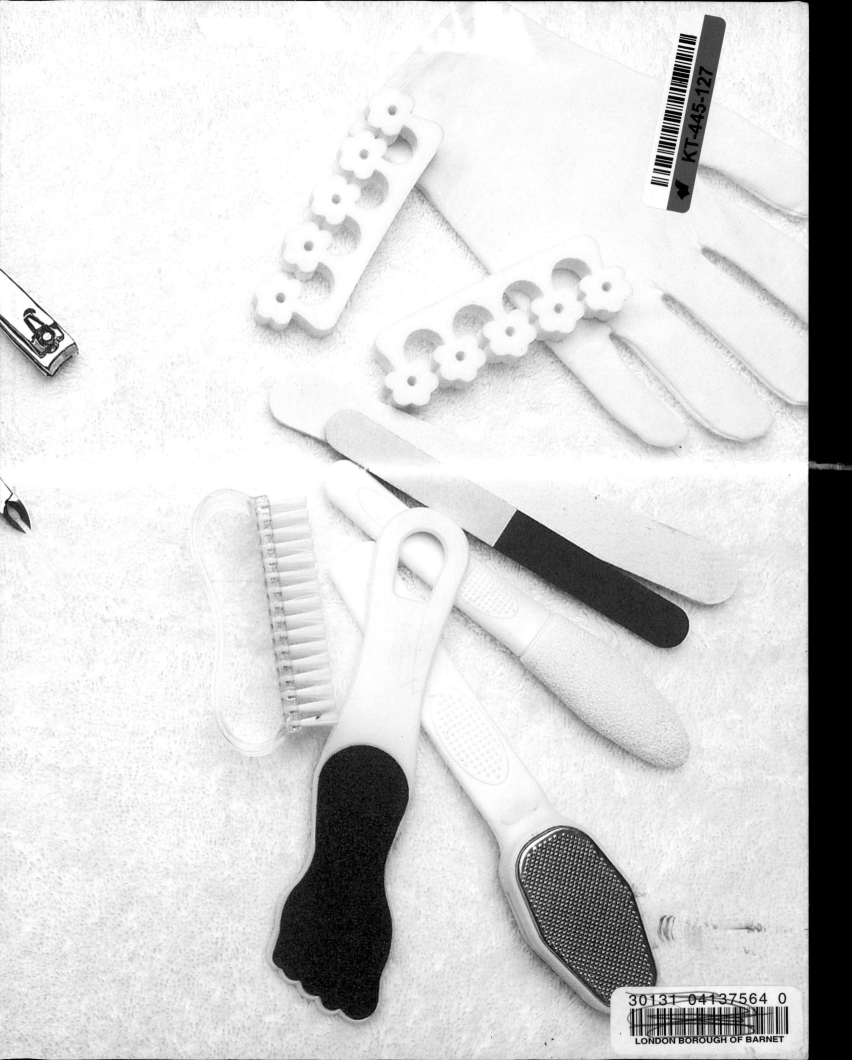

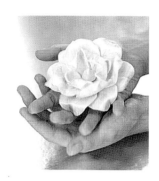

A COMPLETE GUIDE TO
MANICURE
& PEDICURE

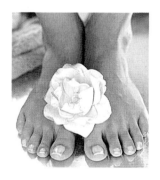

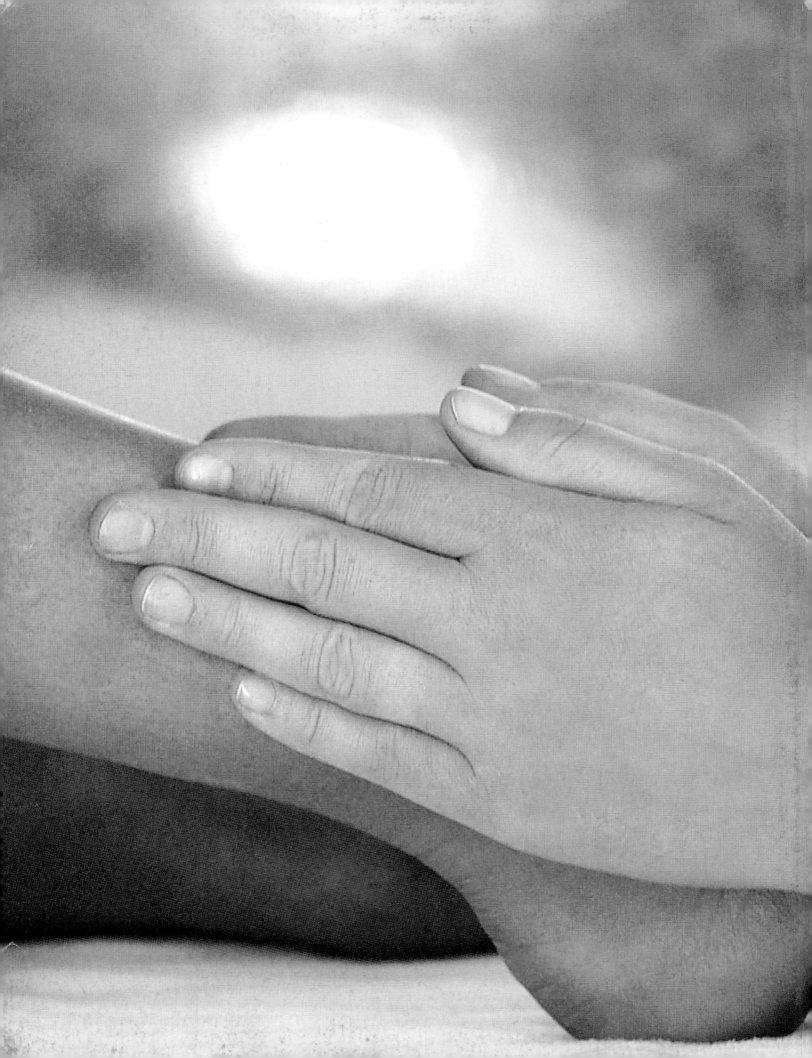

A COMPLETE GUIDE TO
MANICURE
& PEDICURE

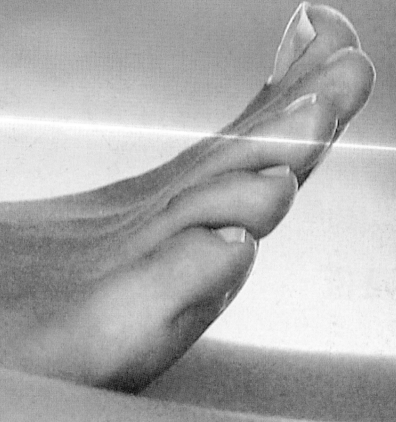

NEW HOLLAND

Leigh Toselli

First published in 2005 by New Holland Publishers Ltd.

London • Cape Town • Sydney • Auckland

• 86 Edgware Road, London, W2 2EA, United Kingdom
• 80 McKenzie Street, Cape Town, 8001, South Africa
• 14 Aquatic Drive, Frenchs Forest, NSW 2086, Australia
• 218 Lake Road, Northcote, Auckland, New Zealand

www.newhollandpublishers.com

NEW
HOLLAND

ISBN (HB) 1 84330 861 4

Publisher: Mariëlle Renssen
Publishing Managers: Claudia Dos Santos, Simon Pooley
Commissioning Editor: Alfred LeMaitre
Studio Manager: Richard MacArthur
Editor: Roxanne Reid
Designer: Lyndall du Toit
Cover Designer: Christelle Marais
Photographer: Patrick Toselli
Illustrator: Louwra Marais
Picture Researcher: Karla Kik
Production: Myrna Collins
Proofreader/indexer: Anna Tanneberger
Consultant: Beryl Barnard FSBTh. M.PHYS. ATT.
   Education Director, The London School of Beauty & Make-up

Reproduction by Resolution Colour (Pty) Ltd., Cape Town, South Africa.
Printed and bound in Singapore by Tien Wah Press (Pte) Ltd.
10 9 8 7 6 5 4 3 2 1

PHOTOGRAPHIC CREDITS

Mediscan: Pg 20 top and bottom; pg 21 right; pg
37 top, bottom left and bottom right; pg 38 top
and bottom; pg 39 top, bottom left, bottom right;
pg 87; pg 89; pg 90 right; pg 92 left and right.

Photofusion: Pg 21 left; pg 84 top right; pg 86.

Images of Africa:
www.imagesofafrica.co.za
(Warren Heath) Pg 31; pg 32; pg 88; pg 97.

Acknowledgements

Grateful thanks to make-up artist Melody Cokayne for her unerring attention to detail, as always; what would we do without you? Also to trainer and nail technician Romilda Britz for translating her work for the camera and for patiently going through each and every step. Thanks, too, to models Daniella and Karolina from G3 Models, and Tamlin and Melanie from Ice Models for allowing us to pretty up their hands and feet – tough job! Leslie Rogers and Stephanus Cronjé also deserve credit for sourcing all the beautiful props and accessories. To Elaine and Stephen Meyer from Viso Bella Skin Care Centre, who are always supportive and accommodating, thanks for allowing us to invade your salon yet again.

I am grateful to Alfred LeMaitre for getting me involved in the first place – I've learnt a lot; to my editor Roxanne Reid for her nurturing, patience and enthusiasm; to Louwra Marais for the illustrations; and to Lyndall du Toit for her wonderful design.

I would also like to acknowledge shoe designer Gianpaulo Bresolin, podiatrist Garyn Cohen, physiotherapist Hilde Kromhout, OPI educator Leana Avent and therapeutic reflexologist Sharon du Raan for answering all my questions.

Thanks for the loan of props and garments go to Dream Nails; Nailene; Estée Lauder; Loads of Living; Foxy; Kookaï; Hadeda; Life Style Emporium; Apsley House; Palazzo Pitti Shoes; Amici Accessories; Accessorize; Crabtree & Evelyn; OPI; Revlon; Nicci Boutique; Green Cross Shoes; and The Body Shop.

Thanks, too, to my mother Delyse Harding for showing us that growing older gracefully is an art and that beautiful hands need lots of TLC; and to my sons Devin, Rowan and Kieran for putting up with my distractions, giving me all their support, and supplying endless cups of tea. And last, but by no means least, a special word of appreciation to my husband Patrick Toselli for his unending support, encouragement and partnership, not to mention his superb photography; where would I be without you?

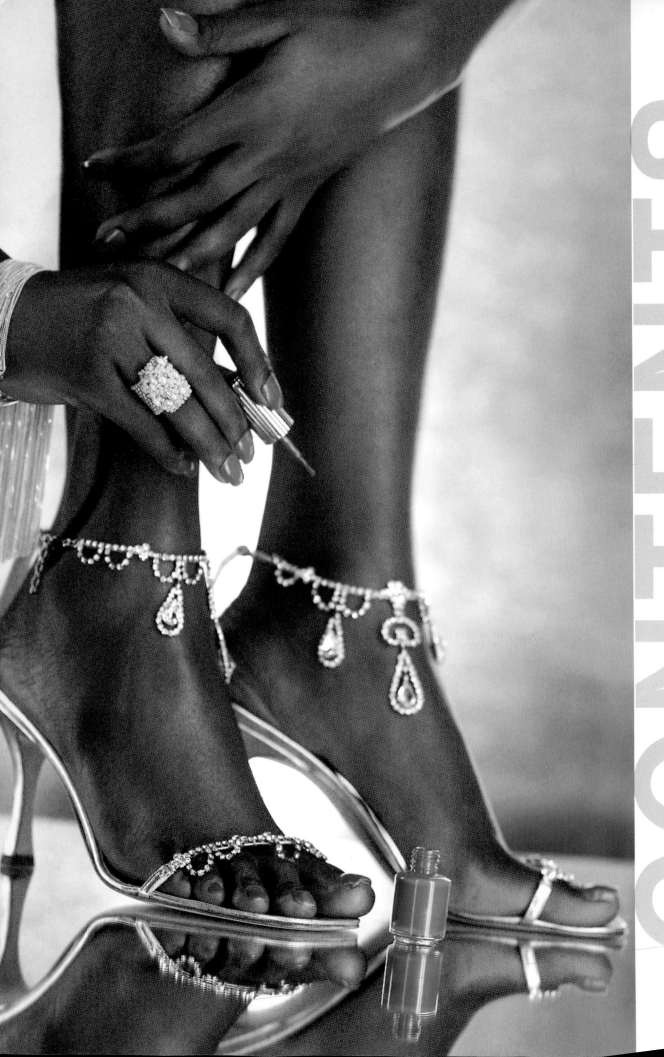

CONTENTS

PART 1 HANDS

PART 2 FEET

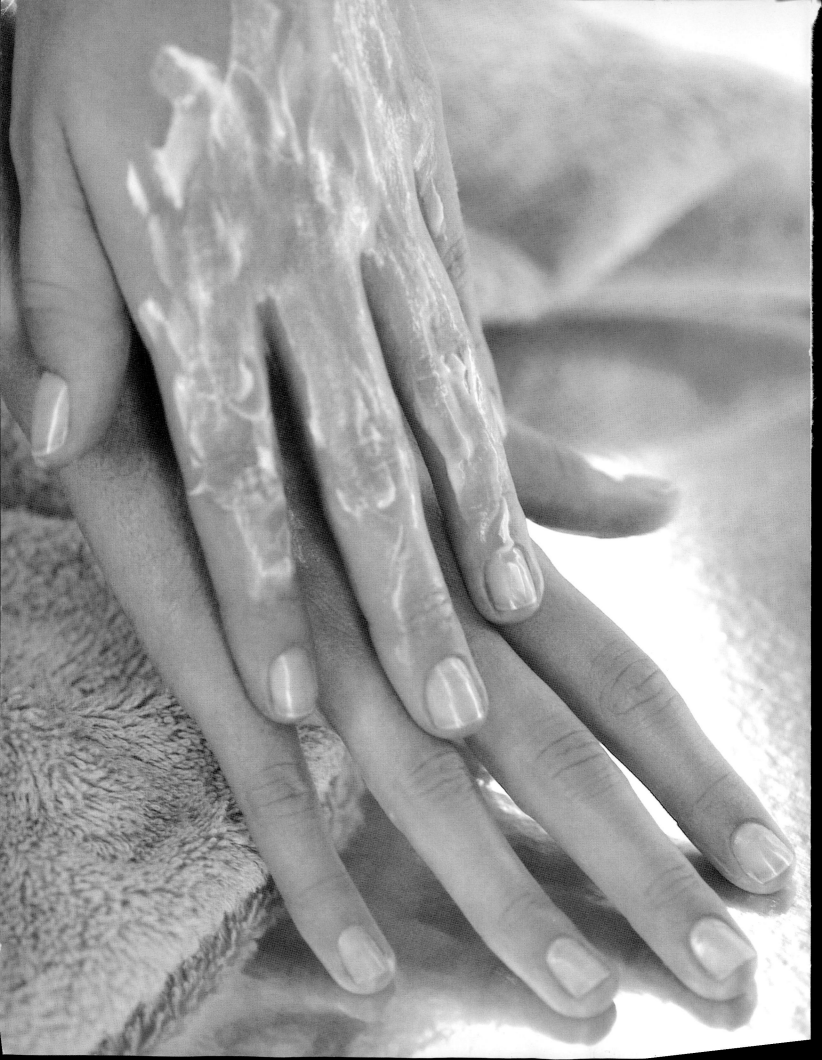

PART ONE

hands

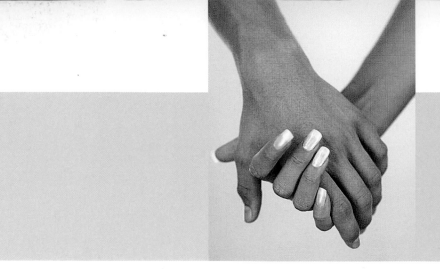

The structure of hands and nails

Graceful, silky hands and beautiful nails are much-prized physical attributes. Supple hands and trim, healthy nails speak volumes about your state of health and personal grooming, whereas neglected hands let the side down; they not only create a poor impression, they belie your age.

We notice each other's hands almost unconsciously because they are used extensively in communication. What impression do your hands make? Do they convey confidence? Bitten nails or torn cuticles are a dead giveaway of a lack of confidence, while hands that are simply and well manicured suggest a person who pays attention to detail and is organized enough to get even the smallest things done.

Your hands are in the front line and bear the brunt of any rough handling, so they deserve care and attention. There is so much that contributes to beautiful hands, but the wonderful aspect of nail technology today is that you no longer need to be genetically programmed to have a beautiful set of nails.

Hand surfaces

Your skin is your first line of defence against the outside world: it warms you, warns other body systems of invaders, and excretes bodily fluids. It is a waterproof, washable and flexible substance that can mend and renew itself. The skin that covers your hands, in particular, functions as a protective shield and is also the focus of your sense of touch.

With rich nerve endings, the skin responds to myriad sensations. Discreetly placed oil glands secrete sebum (a fatty, oily substance) to moisturize and waterproof your skin, while sweat glands excrete toxins to help regulate body heat. Thousands of sensitive nerve endings are embedded in the skin, especially in the finger pads. Ultrasensitive receptors allow you to perceive touch, pressure, warmth and pain, and combinations of these senses expand your perceptions to include ticklishness, wetness and hardness, as well as surface texture, form, force and weight.

The epidermis

The skin comprises three layers. The outermost protective layer is the epidermis. It comprises five layers, including the *stratum corneum*, which is made up of tightly packed, scale-like cells that are constantly being shed and replaced by cells from below as they move to the surface. You lose

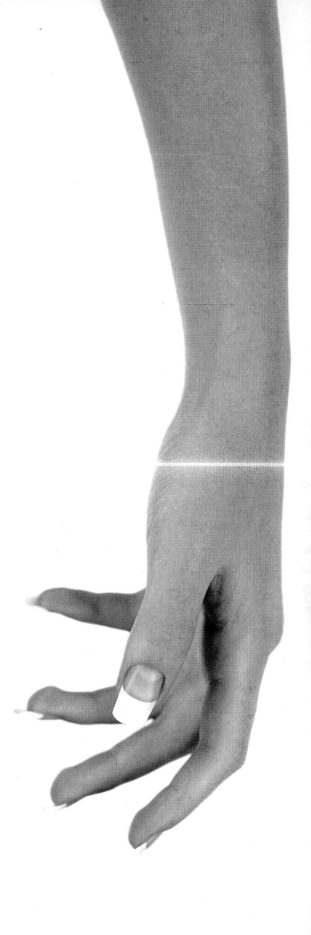

thousands of dead skin cells every time you scratch, rub or wash your hands. The tough cells in this horny layer form a shield that protects the delicate living cells underneath from infection or injury. They contain a waxy, waterproof protein called *keratin*, which makes up skin, nails and hair. A thin coating of oil, or sebum, helps keep the outermost layer pliable, soft and waterproof.

The epidermis is the first line of defence for the body's immune system. With a pH balance of 5.0, it forms an acid shield (mantle) that keeps out harmful substances, protects against injury, dryness and infections, and prevents moisture loss. The epidermis on the palms of the hands and soles of the feet is thicker than elsewhere.

The lowest layer of the epidermis, or basal layer, is where the skin pigment *melanin* is formed by melanocyte cells. Melanin determines the intensity of your particular shade of skin according to your genetic make-up.

Differences in skin colour are the result of the amount, type and arrangement of the melanin in the epidermis. Melanin is designed to absorb ultraviolet rays from the sun, thereby protecting you from its harmful effects, which include ageing, loss of elasticity and pigmentation. The darker your skin colour, the more melanin is present and the better your body can adapt to sun exposure.

The dermis

This is a spongy, closely woven network of connective tissue that is thicker than the epidermis and lies underneath it. It breaks down and renews itself constantly.

Its major components include the proteins *collagen* (for structure)

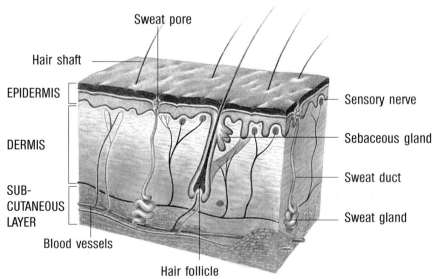

Sweat pore

Hair shaft

EPIDERMIS

DERMIS

SUB-CUTANEOUS LAYER

Blood vessels

Hair follicle

Sensory nerve

Sebaceous gland

Sweat duct

Sweat gland

LAYERS OF SKIN

and *elastin* (for elasticity). Tough protein fibres in the dermis give the skin its tensile strength and bulk. The dermis also contains scattered blood vessels, lymph vessels, nerve endings, hair follicles and glands connected with the epidermis. It is directly connected to the nervous system, glands that produce sebum and sweat, lymph vessels, and 25 per cent of the body's blood supply.

Thousands of tiny projections called *papillae* jut up from the dermis into microscopic pits in the bottom of the epidermis. Papillae grouped in rows form the ridges on your fingers, giving you a distinctive set of fingerprints (*see* page 14). Each papilla has a rich supply of tiny capillaries, or blood vessels, that bring nourishment to growing skin and regulate heat loss from your body. Papillae also contain nerve endings that are sensitive to touch.

Subcutaneous layer

Situated beneath the epidermis and dermis is the third of the skin's primary layers – a protective layer of fat that also contains large blood vessels.

The back of the hand

The skin on the back of your hand, called the *dorsal* skin, is pliable and easily pinched or pulled away from the underlying tissue. Without this suppleness, your fingers would be unable to flex and move. Notice the fine, soft hairs on the back of your hand – about 15 to 20 hairs per square centimetre. These are important as protective warning devices; when hairs are bent, follicles on the skin's surface activate sensitive touch receptors.

The palm

Rich in sensory receptors, and supplied with sweat glands to help lower your body's temperature and eliminate toxins, the skin on the palm of your hand is thick and hairless. It is usually referred to as *volar* skin. This skin is not as flexible as the skin on the back of your hand and is more tightly connected.

Sweat glands in the palms lubricate the skin, enhancing your ability to touch and grasp objects.

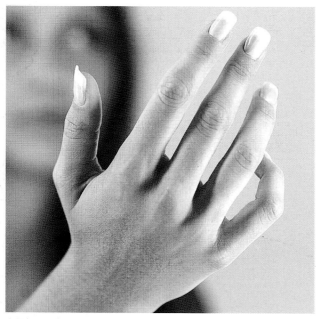

Above: Skin on the back of the hand is thin and pliable. Right: Palmistry uses the fleshy mounts on the palm to indicate character traits.

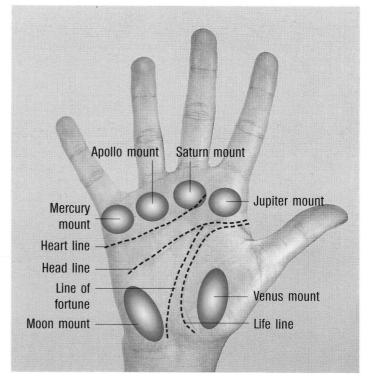

Apollo mount
Saturn mount
Mercury mount
Jupiter mount
Heart line
Head line
Line of fortune
Venus mount
Moon mount
Life line

HAND READING

Through your hand movements, you tell others a great deal about yourself, without always being aware of the messages you are communicating. In addition, the hands have also long been thought of as a symbolic link between the psyche and the soul. The ancient mystical art of palmistry, believed to have been brought to Europe from Asia by gypsies during the Renaissance, attempts to predict a person's destiny by reading the features of the hand.

In palmistry, the fleshy parts of the palm at the base of the thumb and fingers of the hands are called mounts. These are named after Apollo (the god of the sun in Greek mythology), the moon, and the planets Venus, Jupiter, Saturn, Mercury and Mars. A well-developed fleshy mount is supposed to mean that a person has the characteristics associated with that mount. For instance, the mount of Apollo indicates art and riches, Jupiter signifies ambition and pride, and Venus represents love and music.

The wrinkles in the palm are called lines, each with a name and meaning. For example, a long line of life apparently foretells a long life, whereas a long, clear line of the heart indicates an affectionate nature. A strongly marked line of the head is said to signify intelligence and imagination.

Some palmists use the form of the hand to indicate an individual's personality as part of the process of predicting the future. Such signs may help the palmist make surprisingly accurate readings.

The condition of the hands and nails also indicates some characteristics. For example, square fingertips and squared-off nails may indicate common sense, while tapered fingers and oval nails may be associated with idealism. Thin fingers and long, delicate nails can signal an individualist with an anxious temperament, whereas short fingers and broad nails may identify an impulsive nature.

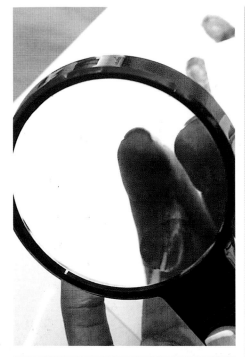

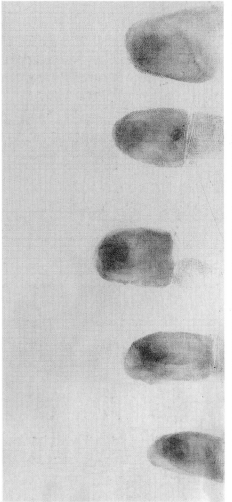

FINGERPRINT PATTERNS

Fingerprints consist of patterns formed by the ridges that are separated by grooves and furrows and cover the skin of the fingertips. Although they provide the most reliable form of identification as no two person's prints are the same, identification is not the only reason for their existence. If your fingertip skin were highly polished and smooth, your capacity for tactile sensation would be greatly reduced .

This imprinted part of your skin has no hairs or sebaceous glands to impede contact with the surface, making them perfectly adapted for touch. Human fingertips are an incredible repository of sensory nerves. They are corrugated and dotted with sweat glands, and have as many as 18 sweat pores per millimetre. This helps lubricate the skin, keeping fingertips supple and enhancing your ability to grasp and touch. As you touch objects with your fingertips, the rough ridges, along with your sensory nerves, create friction between your hand and the object, which helps to improve your perception of temperature, texture and solidity.

There are four main types of fingerprint patterns. In a *loop pattern*, which is the most common type, the ridges begin at one side of the finger, curve back sharply, and end on the same side. The ridges in a *whorl pattern* have a circular form. In an *arch pattern*, the ridges extend from one side of the finger to the other, rising in the centre. An *accidental pattern*, as the name suggests, has no specific form. Many fingerprints combine loops, whorls and arches.

Here are some fascinating fingerprint facts:

- No two people have identical fingerprints.
- Fingerprints begin to form in the second or third month of the life of a foetus.
- Each fingertip has a different pattern, and even the corresponding fingertips on an individual's left and right hands do not match.
- Fingerprints do change in size as you mature but the patterns never change.
- If you injure the tip of a finger, the pattern will return once the finger is healed.

Hand structure

Bones

Anatomically the bones of the hand can be divided into three parts:

- The *carpus*, or wrist, is a flexible joint composed of eight small bones held together by ligaments. The bones of the hand are connected to those of the lower arm by tendons.
- The *metacarpus*, or palm, is the main part of the hand and has five long metacarpal bones.
- The *phalanges*, or fingers, are formed by 14 phalangeal bones. Each finger has three phalanges whereas the thumb has only two.

This complex framework of bones allows a range of fine and gross movements in your hands, which can perform huge tasks, as well as the most delicate and precise functions.

Muscles

The hand has many small muscles that overlap from joint to joint, giving flexibility and strength. When the hands are properly cared for, these muscles will remain supple and graceful.

Abductors separate the fingers and *adductors* draw the fingers together. Both of these types of muscles are located at the base of the thumb and fingers. *Opponent* muscles in the palm of the hand bring the thumb toward the fingers, giving rise to the grasping action of the hand.

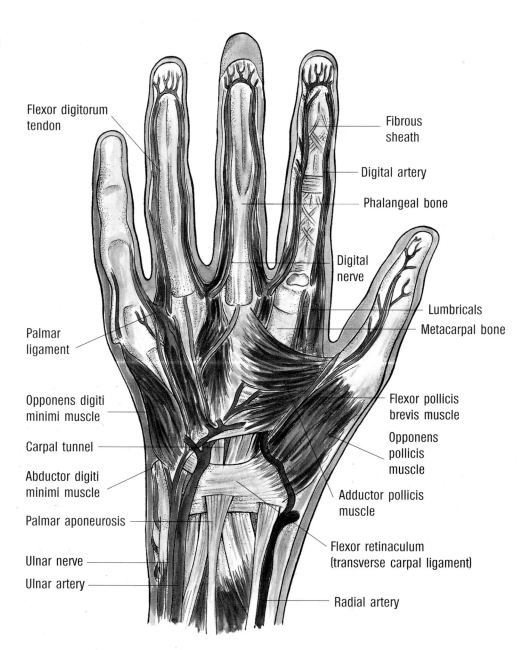

Flexor digitorum tendon

Fibrous sheath

Digital artery

Phalangeal bone

Digital nerve

Palmar ligament

Lumbricals

Metacarpal bone

Opponens digiti minimi muscle

Carpal tunnel

Abductor digiti minimi muscle

Palmar aponeurosis

Ulnar nerve

Ulnar artery

Flexor pollicis brevis muscle

Opponens pollicis muscle

Adductor pollicis muscle

Flexor retinaculum (transverse carpal ligament)

Radial artery

STRUCTURE OF THE PALM OF THE HAND

Nerves

Three major nerves in the hand allow you to feel sensation, experience motion and participate in fine, delicate movement.

The *median nerve* is the main nerve for precision grip; it controls finger flexion (bending fingers into the palm) and wrist flexion (bending the wrist down). It also controls sensation in the palm-side surface of the thumb, index and middle fingers, and half of the ring finger. In addition, it supplies stimulus to the muscles that bring the thumb toward the fingers to enable you to grasp an object.

The *ulnar nerve* works with the median nerve to innervate the muscles responsible for the fine movements of the hand, such as typing, writing or sewing.

The third major nerve, the *radial nerve,* supplies sensation to the back of the hand, affecting the muscles that extend the arm, forearm, hand and fingers.

Muscles, tendons and ligaments

The muscles of the hand cannot work alone but function as an interactive group, together with ligaments and tendons, which consist of tough elastic and connective tissue.

Ligaments are dense fibrous bands that provide stability and connect one bone to another, while still allowing some movement and providing guidance, co-ordination and restraint.

Tendons connect muscle to bone; when the muscle contracts, the strong, cable-like tendon pulls the bone to which it is attached.

All normal movements are balanced between the opposing forces of each of the muscles.

There are 20 small muscle groups for independent finger movements, plus an extra 14

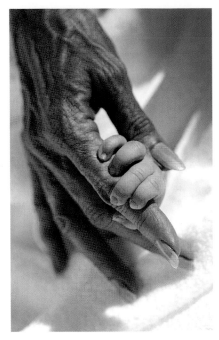

Our hands – complex structures of bones, muscles and nerves – are vital tools throughout our lives.

muscle groups in the forearm. Nine muscles contribute to the flexibility and movement of the thumb, allowing it greater mobility and range of movement than the other fingers as it requires more strength in order to oppose the pressure exerted by four fingers.

The muscle groups in the hands are joined by more than 20 long tendons, which enter the hand under a larger 'wristband' tendon and go forward to form a criss-cross pattern around each finger.

Every muscle, tendon, ligament, nerve and blood vessel is surrounded by connective tissue, which consists of bundles of collagen and elastin. These bundles have three major functions: to

separate or connect structures; to cushion and protect; and to help maintain the shape of the hands, palms and fingers.

Circulatory system

Oxygen and nutrients are transported in the blood to the tissues of the hand by a complex network of arteries, veins and capillaries.

Nutrient- and oxygen-rich blood is carried from your heart through the *brachial artery* of the upper arm and then through either the *radial* or *ulnar arteries,* which carry the main blood supply for the hand and arm. The ulnar artery and its branches supply the outer side of the arm and the palm of the hand, while the radial artery and its branches supply the inner side of the arm and the back of the hand.

Any blockage in the arteries affects your circulation and may result in swelling and pain, or even a mottled, blue or pale discoloration of the hands.

Nails: composition and structure

Your nails serve several purposes: to support the tissues of the fingers and toes; to protect the upper surface of the fingertips from injury; to assist you in picking up small objects; and to help you to grasp, scratch and pinch. Nails also provide external stability to the softer skin that is found around the fingertip.

Your nails are made up of several components – some visible, others not. Their basic ingredient is *keratin*, a fibrous protein that gives nails their tough, hard quality. Keratin is also responsible for human hair, the claws of animals, the horn of a rhinoceros, and the feathers and beaks of birds.

Nails are translucent, usually a faint pinkish colour due to the network of blood vessels beneath them. This colour varies and may lighten when you are cold and the blood vessels become constricted.

Parts of the nail

Half-moon

The whitish, half-moon visible at the base of your nail is the *lunula*. Its pale appearance arises from the fact that it does not adhere so closely to the underlying tissue. It forms a bridge between the living matrix and the nail plate.

It size, shape and brightness varies from person to person and finger to finger, often being more pronounced on the thumb.

Nail matrix

Nail growth begins in the nail *matrix*. Also known as the nail root, it is the living part of the nail hidden under the cuticle. Nail keratin is created here. The matrix contains nerves, lymph vessels and blood vessels vital for nourishing the fingernails. Nail cells divide in the matrix, lengthening the nail plate and pushing it forwards over the nail bed.

Nail bed and nail plate

The most visible part of the nail is called the nail plate – a hard, smooth, slightly convex covering to the fingertip. This is the part we usually think of as the fingernail.

The nail bed is the finger tissue directly under the nail plate; its network of small blood vessels provides nutrition to the nail. While the nail bed supports the nail, it does not contribute to nail growth. As keratin forms in the nail matrix, it pushes forward onto the nail bed to harden and become the exposed nail plate.

The tough nail plate is no longer living tissue, nor does it contain any of the nerves or blood vessels that can be found in the nail bed.

Nail fold

This is the layer of skin covering the edge of the nail plate on all sides except the tip, holding the nail in place. It is usually where nail fungus infections occur.

Cuticle

The cuticle is the thin tissue that grows from the finger to overlap and protect the nail plate and form a rim around the base of the nail. It is the most important part of the nail, protecting both the nail matrix with its delicate tissues and the cells below the nail plate, which are actively forming the hard nail.

Its purpose is to protect against debris, micro-organisms and bacteria that can damage the matrix and nail bed.

Gentleness is the key to cuticle care, as vigorous trimming or pushing back of the cuticles, as well as chemical solvents, may cause ridges in the nail.

In addition, you need to be aware that once the cuticle is damaged, the watertight space under the nail fold is laid open to moisture and becomes a potential breeding ground for bacteria, which can lead to a number of unwanted infections.

FINGERNAIL STRUCTURE

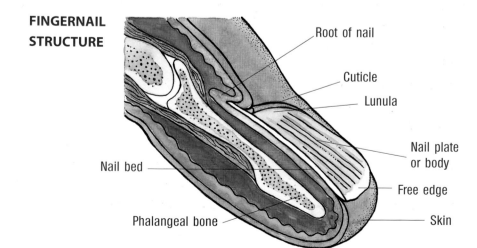

Root of nail
Cuticle
Lunula
Nail plate or body
Free edge
Skin
Nail bed
Phalangeal bone

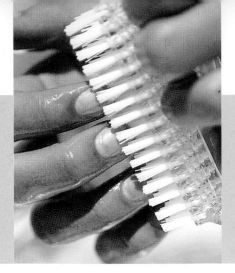

Caring for your hands and nails

When tending to your beauty needs, pay special attention to your hands. Exfoliate them regularly to remove dead skin cells whenever you use a scrub on your body or face. Apply hand cream every time you wash your hands; keep tubs of hand cream handy beside the sink and basin.

Make sure your hand cream includes full-spectrum sunfilters to protect against ultraviolet (UV) radiation. Remember, your hands are continually exposed to the sun's rays – and most ageing, including age spots, is caused by sun damage (*see* box on page 19).

Always wear rubber gloves; plunging unprotected hands and nails into soapy water or household chemicals is like going into the sun without sunscreen. Cotton-lined gloves are best to absorb excess moisture.

THE SUN – your skin's enemy

Sunlight contains ultraviolet (UV) radiation, exposure to which damages cells in your skin. There are three wavelengths of UV light: UVA, UVB and UVC. Chronic exposure to UVA damages your skin and plays a role in both ageing and skin cancer. Sunlight also contains a smaller amount of UVB, which causes sunburn. Although UVC has the potential to injure skin, it does not get the chance as it is absorbed above the earth by the ozone layer.

Photoageing of the skin – responsible for rough, leathery texture, age spots, sagging skin and brown, pigmented freckles on the backs of the hands – is caused by unnecessary and incidental exposure to the sun. Long-term sun exposure also degrades the collagen and elastin structures of the skin, making it less flexible. For all these reasons, it is crucial to apply sunscreen on your hands every day. Check the label to ensure that the sunscreen you choose contains ingredients that filter out both UVA and UVB rays.

Another good idea is to massage your hands with hand cream whenever you have a few spare moments. Use the first finger and the thumb of the opposite hand

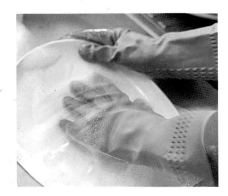

Right: Use gloves to protect hands and nails from harmful chemicals.

and work in small circles, moving from tips of fingers to wrist. (For more about massage techniques, *see* pages 78–79.) Finger exercises can prevent Occupational Overuse Syndrome (*see* page 22), which occurs from constant, repetitive actions, such as typing. Exercise your fingers by clenching them into a ball, then slowly releasing them and stretching the fingers out. Rotate your wrists in circular movements.

8 STEPS TO HEALTHY HANDS

1 **Eat right. Choose foods that are healthy and as close to natural as possible. Vary the type of fruit and vegetables you eat.**

2 **Drink at least six glasses of pure water a day to keep the skin moisturized inside and out.**

3 **Get the sleep your body needs – usually six to eight hours.**

4 **Wear sunscreen and protective clothing to avoid over-exposing your skin to the elements. Some sunshine is necessary but today's suntan is tomorrow's ageing skin.**

5 **Avoid temperature extremes and harsh detergents – rather wash with mild cleansers. As a normal skin function, sweat and sebaceous glands routinely rid the body of toxins and wastes.**

6 **Protect your hands with moisturizing creams, sunscreen or the appropriate gloves when exposing your hands to abrasive or environmental elements.**

7 **Before you go to sleep, rub a rich hand cream or petroleum jelly into hands and nails, massaging around cuticles to mourish and stimulate growth. Then cover with an old pair of cotton gloves. Keep the gloves on overnight, allowing the heat of your hands to work with the moisturizer to provide a 'hot-oil' style treatment.**

8 **Exercise. When faced with repetitive tasks, take time out to stretch and wiggle your fingers, wrists, hands and arms to maintain normal range of movement. (See page 23 for some useful finger exercises.)**

Skin ailments

The skin on the fingers, hands and arms is prone to many problems, from allergies to warts. These are some of the most common:

Itching
Generalized itching may be an allergic reaction to a medication, cosmetic or skin-care product. Apply cold compresses and see a dermatologist to track down the source. (Note, too, that if your eyelids are itchy, you may have a contact allergy to the formaldehyde in the polish on your nails. Switch to a formaldehyde-free formula.)

Rough, chapped hands
These may be caused by exposure to cold weather or by repeatedly washing your hands with harsh detergents, which may further contribute to cracks and fissures. Dry, chapped skin may also be an early sign of vitamin A deficiency. Use gloves when washing dishes, avoid over-washing and harsh detergents, and moisturize your hands regularly.

Eczema
Eczema is a form of dermatitis characterized by inflammation of the skin, with redness, pain or itching. Blisters may develop, and sometimes break, scale and crust over. The causes are legion, including allergies, irritation, extreme dryness, stress and genetic factors. If caused by a reaction to certain

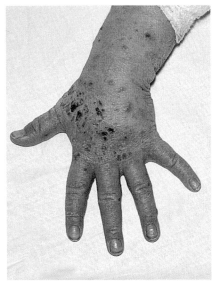

ECZEMA

substances that touch the skin, harsh detergents, chemicals and poisonous plants are often the culprits, so should be avoided. If severe, consult a dermatologist.

Allergies
Skin can be adversely affected by cosmetics, clothing, chemicals, air pollution, not to mention changes in your health or diet. Reactions appear as allergic swelling, hives, blemishes, rashes or local irritation. The best way to handle contact allergies – which are the most likely to affect your hands – is to avoid the offending substance, so protect yourself by being aware of what you touch.

Remember, too, that you may have contact with an allergen and the allergic reaction shows up in another area of your body, so wearing gloves is the best defence.

Warts
Warts are small, hard abnormal growths on the skin caused by a viral infection in the top layer of the skin or mucous membranes. They belong to the *papillomavirus* group. Wart viruses are spread by touch but it can take several months before the wart becomes big enough to be visible.

Warts are usually skin-coloured and rough-textured, though some of them can also be dark, smooth and flat. Most warts will eventually disappear but be aware that scratching and picking will cause them to spread and should therefore be avoided.

Talk to your pharmacist about an over-the-counter preparation and if this does not work, be sure to seek medical help.

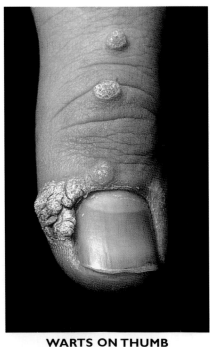

WARTS ON THUMB

Joint problems

Arthritis

Arthritis causes cartilage to degenerate and the bones to become overgrown or waste away. It attacks the linings of the joints, which become stiff, swollen and painful. Muscles that move the joints are unable to work correctly and they waste away, while tissues around the joints become inflamed, filled with fluid – not to mention painful.

The two common forms of arthritis are osteoarthritis and rheumatoid arthritis.

Osteoarthritis is a degenerative joint disease in which the protective, shock-absorbing cartilage between the bones of the joint wears away. It is aggravated by impaired blood supply, previous injury, or by being overweight.

Rheumatoid arthritis, a progressive, destructive swelling of the joints, is usually of unknown origin, though it may be a virus infection. Often affecting the elderly, this incapacitating condition is more common among women. It may be triggered by emotional stress. People suffering from this auto-immune disorder are more susceptible than others to infection.

It can be debilitating, but regular exercise can help build muscle tone. Though exercising a hot, inflamed joint is not advisable, try to move the hand through its full range of movement at least once a day to maintain mobility. Applying heat can ease pain and reduce muscle spasms.

The essential fatty acid omega-3 helps reduce inflammation, so make omega-3-rich fish (mackerel, freshwater trout, tuna, salmon and herring) a regular part of your diet.

Gout

This metabolic disease is associated with excess uric acid in the blood and the deposit of uric acid salts around the joints. It is characterized by painful inflammation and swelling of the small joints, but tends to favour the big toe. It usually affects men, and is perhaps triggered by emotional stress.

Avoid or cut down on red meats, offal, shellfish (mussels and oysters), peas, beans and alcohol, especially beer and wine.

For immediate relief, anti-inflammatory medication can be effective, but seek medical advice in the early stages.

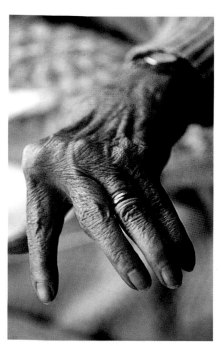

ARTHRITIS

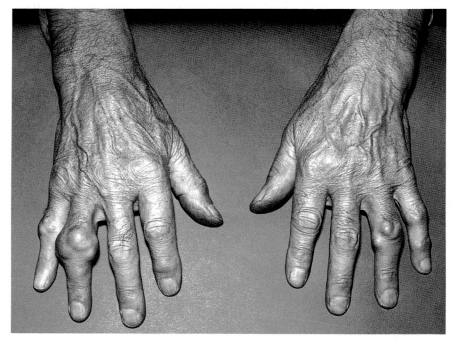

GOUT

Flexibility and movement

Whether typing or swinging a tennis racquet, human fingers, wrists and arms are designed for movement. With time and over-use, however, all of us are affected by the stiffness and aches resulting from overuse.

Occupational Overuse Syndrome (OOS) – also known as *Repetitive Strain Injury (RSI)* – is the term given to a range of conditions characterized by discomfort or persistent pain in muscles, tendons and other soft tissues. These are usually caused or aggravated by unsuitable working conditions involving repetitive or forceful movements, or by maintaining constrained or awkward postures, such as those experienced by musicians and factory workers.

Symptoms often include swelling, numbness, restricted movement and weakness in or around muscles and tendons of the back, neck, shoulders, elbows, wrists, hands or fingers. It may become difficult to hold objects or tools in the hands, affecting your ability to function at work and at home.

Some of the problems that can be caused by OOS include:

Carpal Tunnel Syndrome: This is pressure on the median nerve in the wrist, which causes pain, numbness and tingling in the thumb, index finger and middle

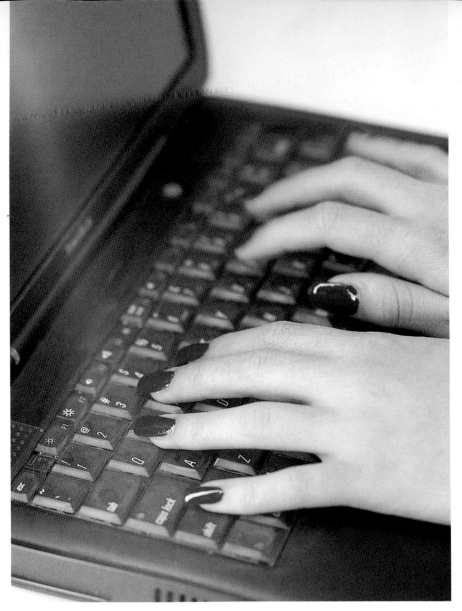

The static hand position and repetitiveness of typing can lead to strain.

finger of the affected hand. The condition mainly affects people who use their fingers a lot, such as typists, housewives or pianists. The pain tends to be worse at night, gradually getting worse over a period of weeks. Try to avoid movements that cause pain and consult a doctor.

Tenosynovitis: This is characterized by pain and swelling of the tendons, often in hands and wrists.

Epicondylitis: This condition is accompanid by pain and tenderness of the muscles and tendons around the elbow. It is commonly referred to as tennis elbow, but caused by any repetitive motion.

Static Muscle Strain: This occurs when muscles are used to keep part of the body still and stiff for long periods, causing pain and stiffness in muscles, often in the shoulders, neck and forearm.

Hand and finger exercises

Most of us will be affected at some point by stiffness and aches resulting from overuse of our joints. Try taking a break from repetitive tasks, and stretch your hands and arms several times to relieve tension.

In fact, exercising your hands and fingers is important in order to maintain flexibility and movement. Here are some simple exercises you can do each morning to tone and stretch your arm muscles, boost circulation and limber up your joints for the day ahead.

1 Fist fling: Clench both fists tightly, hold for a second, throw open the fingers, forward and as wide as possible. Repeat six times.

A 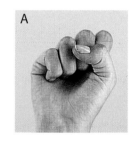 B 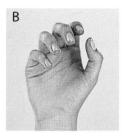 C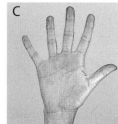

2 Finger spread: Hold your hands straight in front of you, palms down, fingers pressed tightly against each other. Now thrust your fingers apart, opening as wide as possible. Repeat six times.

A 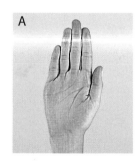 B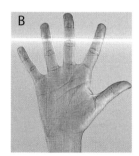

3 Hand circles: Keeping your hands limp and relaxed, rotate them from the wrist in circles, first in one direction, then the other. Rotate 10 times in each direction.

A 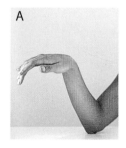 B 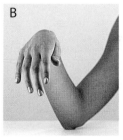 C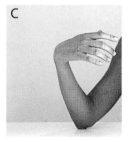

4 Vertical lift: Holding your hands gracefully, palms down, lift up slowly from the wrist, then drop wrist down. Keep the hands very relaxed, but not absolutely limp. Repeat 10 times.

A 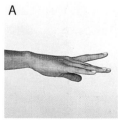 B 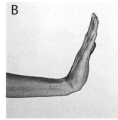 C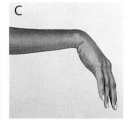

Hand reflexology

Worry beads, rosaries, buttons ... manipulating things with our hands has always been a method of relieving stress. Other alternatives are to use chrome stress balls to exercise the hands, wrists and forearms, or to try some on-the-spot reflexology for rapid relief.

Most people have heard about reflexology on the feet (see pages 124–125), but few know that hand reflexology is just as good, and even quicker for those who cannot sit still. You can do it anytime, anywhere. Once you know which part of the hand to work on, you can relieve specific health complaints, as well as bring your body's energy flow back into balance, which is the ultimate aim.

Reflexology works by stimulating certain points on the hands and feet; this, in turn, stimulates the flow of vital energy, or *chi*, that flows between our internal organs. The theory is that if this energy is blocked or stagnated, the body cannot heal itself and becomes unbalanced.

Reflexology can remove energy blockages in all areas of the body by increasing circulation, removing tension and detoxifying. Once energy is flowing freely again, the body can heal itself and stay strong and healthy.

Hand reflexology is a useful alternative when your feet are muffled in winter layers. It is also much easier than foot reflexology for a DIY treatment as you can easily reach all the reflex points. After all, it is not ideal to sit twiddling your toes at your desk, but you can help a headache by rubbing the tips of your fingers even while having a face-off with your boss. If you have a chronic condition or are pregnant, however, see a professional.

One drawback of hand reflexology is that the structure of the hand, with its small bones and very little flesh, makes it less satisfying than a foot rub.

Theoretically, the right hand mirrors the right side of the body with its organs, including the liver, while the left hand is home to the heart reflex point and a reflex point that stimulates the spleen. The spleen makes and stores red blood cells, and produces the infection-fighting part of the immune system. Stimulate by rotating the tip of the left index finger in a clockwise direction, pressing down on your hand.

Try these reflexology techniques for specific complaints:

Back pain: Use the thumb of the right hand to walk up and down one side of the thumb (A/B) on the left hand and then the other side (C) – see opposite above right. Repeat on the other hand. Repeat the movement every hour for three days, continuing until the problem clears.

Sinusitis: Use your thumb to walk up the fingers on the palm side of each hand. Do this every 40 minutes until you feel relief. After that, use the technique whenever sinusitis is present.

Nervous tension: Massage the web area between your thumb and index finger on each hand.

Insomnia: Gently massage the solar plexus reflex point, which is found on the side of each hand below the index finger and just above the web area.

Left: Worry beads can be useful to exercise your hands and relieve tension.

Hand and finger exercises

Most of us will be affected at some point by stiffness and aches resulting from overuse of our joints. Try taking a break from repetitive tasks, and stretch your hands and arms several times to relieve tension.

In fact, exercising your hands and fingers is important in order to maintain flexibility and movement. Here are some simple exercises you can do each morning to tone and stretch your arm muscles, boost circulation and limber up your joints for the day ahead.

1 **Fist fling:** Clench both fists tightly, hold for a second, throw open the fingers, forward and as wide as possible. Repeat six times.

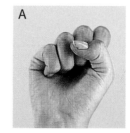 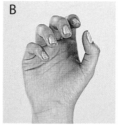 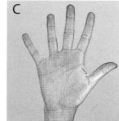

2 **Finger spread:** Hold your hands straight in front of you, palms down, fingers pressed tightly against each other. Now thrust your fingers apart, opening as wide as possible. Repeat six times.

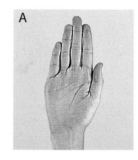 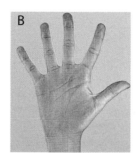

3 **Hand circles:** Keeping your hands limp and relaxed, rotate them from the wrist in circles, first in one direction, then the other. Rotate 10 times in each direction.

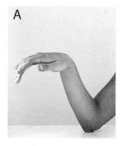 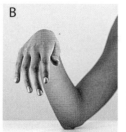 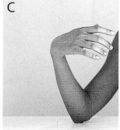

4 **Vertical lift:** Holding your hands gracefully, palms down, lift up slowly from the wrist, then drop wrist down. Keep the hands very relaxed, but not absolutely limp. Repeat 10 times.

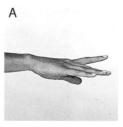 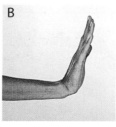 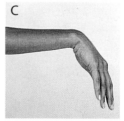

Hand reflexology

Worry beads, rosaries, buttons … manipulating things with our hands has always been a method of relieving stress. Other alternatives are to use chrome stress balls to exercise the hands, wrists and forearms, or to try some on-the-spot reflexology for rapid relief.

Most people have heard about reflexology on the feet (*see* pages 124–125), but few know that hand reflexology is just as good, and even quicker for those who cannot sit still. You can do it anytime, anywhere. Once you know which part of the hand to work on, you can relieve specific health complaints, as well as bring your body's energy flow back into balance, which is the ultimate aim.

Reflexology works by stimulating certain points on the hands and feet; this, in turn, stimulates the flow of vital energy, or *chi*, that flows between our internal organs. The theory is that if this energy is blocked or stagnated, the body cannot heal itself and becomes unbalanced.

Reflexology can remove energy blockages in all areas of the body by increasing circulation, removing tension and detoxifying. Once energy is flowing freely again, the body can heal itself and stay strong and healthy.

Hand reflexology is a useful alternative when your feet are muffled in winter layers. It is also much easier than foot reflexology for a DIY treatment as you can easily reach all the reflex points. After all, it is not ideal to sit twiddling your toes at your desk, but you can help a headache by rubbing the tips of your fingers even while having a face-off with your boss. If you have a chronic condition or are pregnant, however, see a professional.

One drawback of hand reflexology is that the structure of the hand, with its small bones and very little flesh, makes it less satisfying than a foot rub.

Theoretically, the right hand mirrors the right side of the body with its organs, including the liver, while the left hand is home to the heart reflex point and a reflex point that stimulates the spleen. The spleen makes and stores red blood cells, and produces the infection-fighting parts of the immune system. Stimulate it by rotating the tip of the left index finger in a clockwise direction, pressing down on your hand.

Try these reflexology techniques for specific complaints:

Back pain: Use the thumb of the right hand to walk up and down one side of the thumb (A/B) on the left hand and then the other side (C) – *see* opposite above right. Repeat on the other hand. Repeat the movement every hour for three days, continuing until the problem clears.

Sinusitis: Use your thumb to walk up the fingers on the palm side of each hand. Do this every 40 minutes until you feel relief. After this, use the technique whenever sinusitis is present.

Nervous tension: Massage the web area between your thumb and index finger on each hand.

Insomnia: Gently massage the solar plexus reflex point, which is found on the side of each hand below the index finger and just above the web area.

Left: Worry beads can be useful to exercise your hands and relieve tension.

A 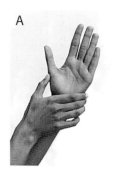 B 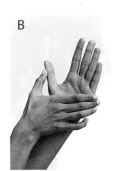 C 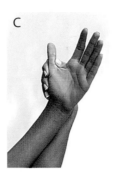 A B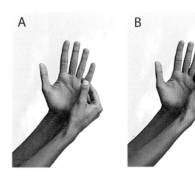

BACK PAIN

SINUSITIS

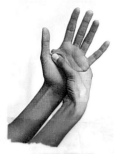

NERVOUS TENSION

THE REFLEXOLOGY HAND CHART

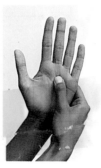

INSOMNIA

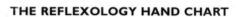

Sinuses

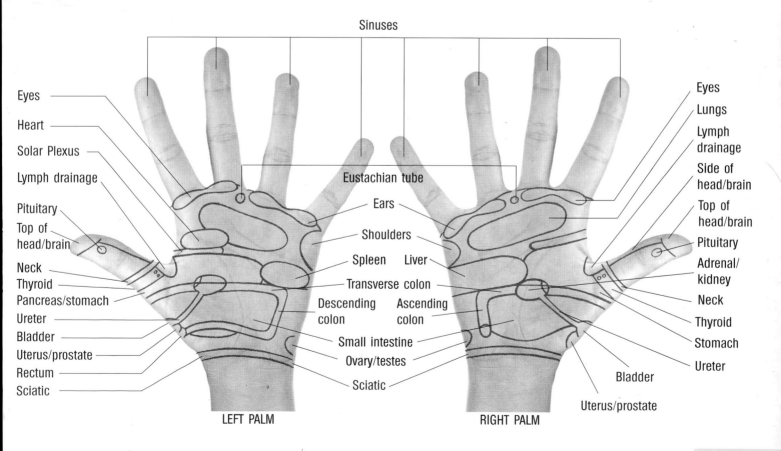

Eyes

Heart

Solar Plexus

Lymph drainage

Pituitary

Top of head/brain

Neck

Thyroid

Pancreas/stomach

Ureter

Bladder

Uterus/prostate

Rectum

Sciatic

Eustachian tube

Ears

Shoulders

Spleen   Liver

Transverse colon

Descending   Ascending
colon   colon

Small intestine

Ovary/testes

Sciatic

Eyes

Lungs

Lymph drainage

Side of head/brain

Top of head/brain

Pituitary

Adrenal/kidney

Neck

Thyroid

Stomach

Ureter

Bladder

Uterus/prostate

LEFT PALM

RIGHT PALM

25

Ageing hands

Hand care should be an integral part of every woman's beauty regime, but women who spend a fortune on age-retarding face creams often seem to forget about their hands. At 40 your face might look 10 years younger, but your hands never lie – age spots begin to appear and one of the first signs of a fading youth is the loose, crepy skin on the backs of your hands.

In many ways your hands mirror and chronicle your life experience. More than any other area of the body, hands are exposed to all sorts of damage; abuse them and they will give away your age.

The age of your skin is partially determined by its content of water-soluble collagen, a protein needed to form connective tissue. It gives skin its flexibility and ability to absorb moisture. As the skin thins and ages, collagen and elastin fibres – the skin's structural support – degenerate. Collagen molecules start to oxidize, becoming stiffer and less able to absorb moisture. This results in the appearance of lines and wrinkles. Sun damage also becomes more visible. Usually, these signs of ageing are first seen around the eyes, on the neck and the backs of your hands as this is where the skin is thinnest. These areas are also the most vulnerable to the cumulative effect of the sun's rays, which speed up the cellular deterioration of the skin.

As you grow older and abuse your hands, your skin loses its elasticity and your hands become more susceptible to brown spots; bruises and black-and-blue marks; calluses; dry, fragile skin; poor bone health; cold hands; and dilated veins. Brown spots (often

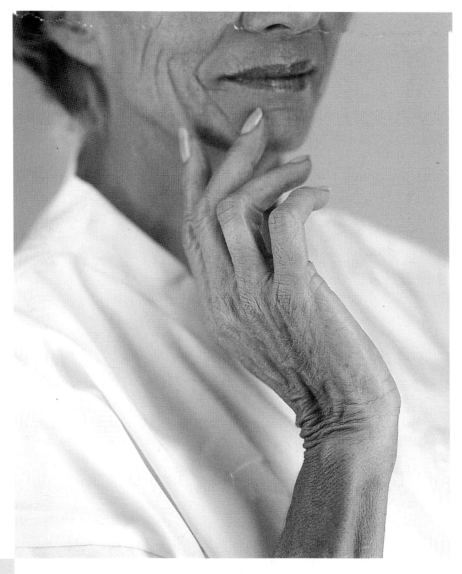

Left: Hands are often the first to give away your age. Retard the effects of ageing with regular use of sunscreen.

incorrectly called 'liver spots') on the back of the hands are the result of the cumulative effects of sunlight or chronic bruising of the skin. These can be retarded, and often prevented, by meticulous use of a full-spectrum sunscreen.

Nails suffer, too. As you age, they become thinner and rougher, often developing ridges due to the natural changes in the matrix, which is responsible for growth.

Healthy nails

Maintaining healthy, natural nails is not as complicated as many may think. As with hair, nails are usually their healthiest in their natural state, requiring a bit of nail polish for protection and regular applications of hand cream to act as a moisturizer.

Frequent nail splitting can indicate dehydration. In such cases, drink more fluids and use an oil designed to penetrate the nail plate. Follow up with regular use of cuticle cream. It will take six months to see results.

Remember that regular long-term use of nail polish can cause a yellowing discoloration of the nails. Although this is not considered damaging, it is useful to know that it can be minimized by always using a basecoat to protect the nails.

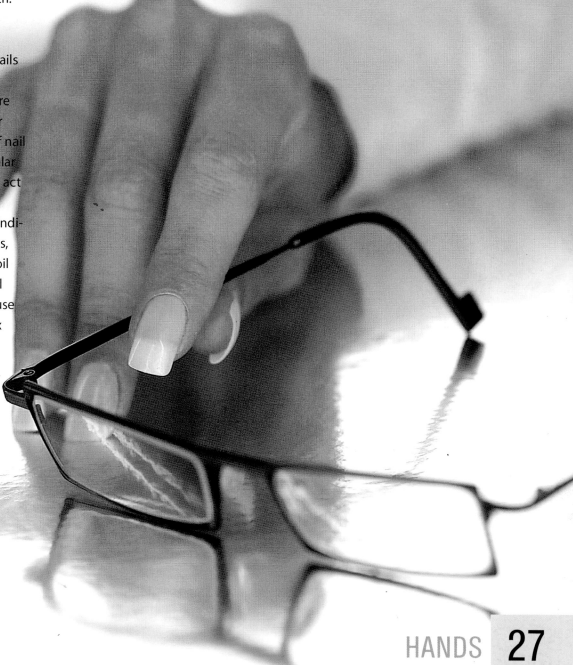

15 NAIL-CARE TIPS

1 Apply a hand cream or lotion after washing your hands as soaps make nails and skin very dry, leading to brittle, peeling nails.

2 Sweet almond oil, combined with a little salt and rubbed into the nails and cuticles, will help to strengthen weak or broken nails, as well as provide nourishment to dry and flaking cuticles.

3 Treat your cuticles very gently as they protect the growth centre of the nail. Never tear the skin or cut the cuticles.

4 Break the habit of nail biting, which can damage the nail and the cuticle, leading to a deformed nail shape or uneven nail growth. (For tips on how to stop biting, see page 34.) Note that biting nails can also transfer harmful organisms to the nail that lead to infection or even increase your chance of catching a cold or flu.

5 Stimulate your nails to encourage growth. Massage the base of your nails whenever you can. Typing, piano playing and any other exercise that requires substantial finger movement will increase the blood supply to the fingers.

6 Unless your nails are very long, avoid clipping to shorten as this can bend or split them. Rather use an emery board to file nails down to size. Filing straight up against your nail can peel the tip, so hold the emery board at a 45-degree angle under the free edge of the nail.

7 After removing your nail polish, wait a few minutes before you start filing to shape or shorten your nails. The nails may split if they are not dry.

8 Use nail polish remover as infrequently as possible, especially those containing acetone, as most will dry nails out. Many specialists suggest using remover no more than once a week. Use a minimal amount of remover on the nail and avoid getting too much on either the cuticle or the surrounding skin.

9 Never scrape off nail polish or use metal instruments to push back cuticles. This can scrape off the protective cells of the nail surface. Peeling off flaking nail enamel can also be very damaging to the nail.

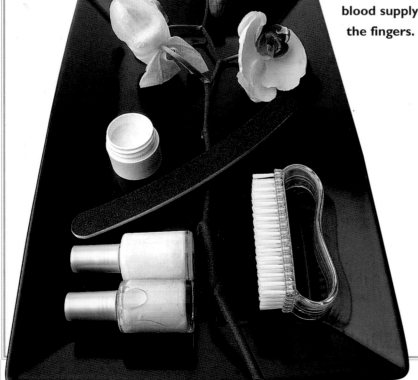

10 **Nail nourishers are quick to apply and pay big beauty dividends by feeding the skin around the nail, as well as the surrounding skin, with essential vitamins, oils and protein. This helps the nails to grow long, strong and healthy.**

11 **Manicure your nails fully every 7–14 days, reapplying nail polish as often as needed to maintain a well-groomed appearance.**

12 **Apply a topcoat almost daily to protect the tips.**

13 **The fastest way to prevent soft, weak nails from breaking is to apply a hardener once or twice a week; it not only saves vulnerable nails but gives a high-shine finish.**

14 **Basecoat is a good investment. Although formulated to help your nail polish last longer, it also helps to prevent bright colour from staining your nails. (A useful tip if your nails are stained is for you to try dipping the tips in half a lemon for 15 seconds. The citric acid in the lemon juice acts as a bleach.**

However, always remember to wash your hands afterward so that the lemon juice does not dry out your hands.)

15 **Nail polish is also a good nail protector. When applying nail polish, especially dark colours, be sure to apply two to three thin coats rather** than a single thick coat. Do not take the polish right to the edges of your nails; it is quicker and much neater to leave a thin strip down each side. It alo makes nails look slimmer. Apply the first stroke of polish along the centre of the nail, then apply polish along the sides in two strokes for a neat finish.

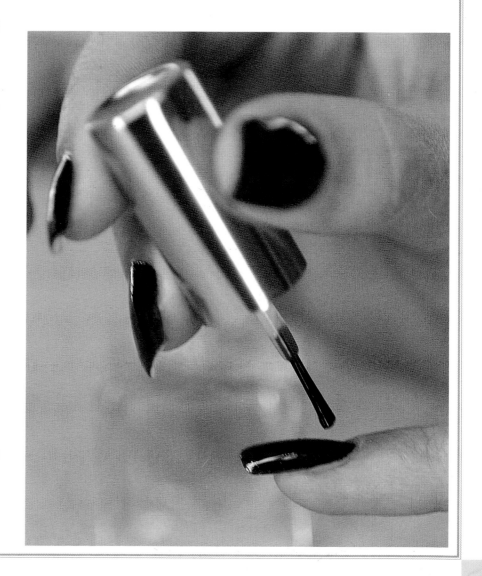

Cuticle care

The cuticle is the thin strip of skin that runs along the base of the nail. Its function is to protect the nail by acting as a barrier against bacteria that may try to work their way under the nail and damage the live cells that are being formed just underneath.

Proper cuticle care is important. Massage your cuticles and nails with cuticle oil, cod liver oil or almond oil to nourish and stimulate growth. Pay special attention to the white half-moon at the base of the nails.

If cuticles are neglected and become dry and you handle them roughly, they could become sore. If you push cuticles back too roughly, you may damage the new cells underneath – and the future growth of your nails. The best time to push back dry or ragged cuticles is right after a bath, when they are soft from the warm water.

Never clip cuticles or chew around them as hangnails (*see* page 36) may develop. Do not pull or tear cuticles. To prevent them from pulling back any further, always cut away gently with nail nippers, leaving the cuticle as intact and untampered with as possible. There is no risk of infection if you sterilize the nippers.

If the cuticle is hard and dry, and sticks up, trim it slightly, but never remove the whole thing. Control strong cuticle growth with a cuticle softener. Apply a little to the cuticle of each nail and massage well into the base of each nail with your fingers to ensure that it works properly. Leave it to work for three minutes, or as long as instructed. Then gently push your cuticles back using a cottonwool-covered hoof stick or orange stick (*see* page 42), or a rubber-tipped cuticle-pusher.

Remove any residue with a tissue. Always remember to rinse your nails in warm water to ensure that they are really clean.

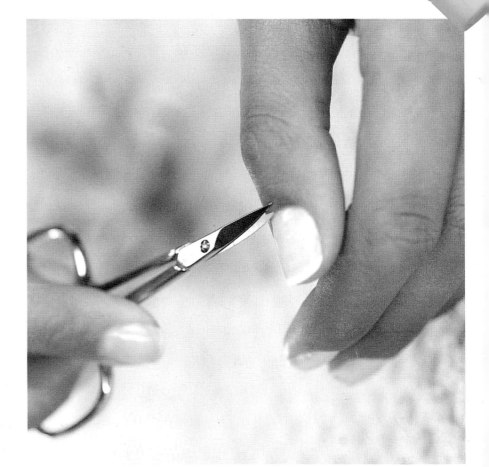

Trim cuticles gently with nail scissors only if they are very hard and dry.

Nail nutrition

The best route to beautiful nails is to follow a healthy, balanced diet of fresh, wholesome food, including vitamin- and mineral-rich foods. Increasing your consumption of fruits and vegetables to five or more servings a day can improve the health of your nails, as well as reduce your risk of chronic and life-threatening diseases such as heart disease and cancer.

Remember, nails grow slowly so it takes a few months before any difference is perceptible. Unless you are severely malnourished, you probably get what your nails need from your daily diet and intake of vitamin supplements. Nail supplements may be overrated as most healthy, westernized diets today contain everything we need; in fact, we generally urinate supplements out of our systems.

Far better to ensure that you eat enough of the right foods. Here is a list of nutrients that contribute to healthy nail growth – and where you can find them:

Vitamin A helps firm thin nails and boost bone growth. Find it in fish, liver, egg yolk, milk, spinach, broccoli and red/yellow vegetables.

Vitamin B7 (biotin) and **vitamin H** have been shown to strengthen nails by aiding nail-cell growth. Good sources are brewer's yeast, broccoli, cheese, nuts, soya, sunflower seeds, sweet potatoes and whole grains.

Vitamin B2 (riboflavin) promotes healthy skin, hair and nails. It is found in carrots, asparagus, spinach, sweet potatoes, apples, garlic, ginger, papaya and high-coloured fruits and vegetables.

Vitamin B12 (cobalamin) helps the body absorb protein, aiding in nail-cell formation. Sources include milk, cheese, eggs, and seaweed such as kelp and nori.

Vitamin C (ascorbic acid) helps prevent hangnails and swelling of nail tissue. Eat fresh fruit (especially citrus), tomatoes, asparagus, red peppers, broccoli, potatoes, nuts, squash, wheatgerm and barley.

Vitamin D (calciferol) enhances absorption of calcium, which prevents dry, brittle nails. Get vitamin D from sunlight on the skin, fish, fish oils, liver and milk.

Vitamin E (tocopherol) helps to prevent yellowed nails and boost circulation. It is found in leafy green vegetables, nuts, seeds and vegetable oils and dairy products.

Calcium contributes to the growth and maintenance of teeth, bones and nails. Good sources include tofu and nuts, bitter leafy greens such as dandelion and broccoli, and dairy products such as milk and cheese.

Fatty acids: flaky, dry nails often respond well to a supplement of evening primrose or starflower oils, which both contain polyunsaturated fatty acids needed to form the structure of cell membranes and lock in moisture.

Iron is an essential nutrient, a deficiency of which can make your nails thin and flat. Increase your intake by eating lean red meat, dark green vegetables, dried fruit and nuts.

Magnesium is important for nail growth. It also stimulates nerve and muscle action. Good sources of magnesium include whole-grain breads and cereals, leafy green vegetables, nuts, beans milk and fish.

Protein is needed for healthy keratin formation. Too little can weaken nails, so make sure that you get your fair share. Eat two portions a day of the following: meat, fish, eggs, cheese or milk. All foods contain protein, even vegetables, fruits and grains, so most people who follow a healthy diet get more than enough each day. (Vegetarians or vegans who are concerned about the state of their nails should increase their intake of dark green leafy veg-etables and flax oil.)

Silicone helps nails to use calcium effectively and is necessary for nail formation. Find it in alfalfa sprouts, brown rice, peppers, soya, and leafy green vegetables, as well as whole grains.

Sulphur accounts for nearly 10 per cent of a healthy body's content and is vital to nail, muscle, hair and skin cells. Make sure you fill up on Brussels sprouts, cabbage, dairy products, eggs, garlic, lean meat and seafood, nuts and seeds, pulses, onions, turnips, wheatgerm and whole grains.

Zinc contributes to cell growth and function and is also an essential nutrient for healthy skin and nails. Good sources of this mineral include brewer's yeast, egg yolks, pulses, pumpkin, pecan nuts, sunflower seeds, wheat bran, and whole grains.

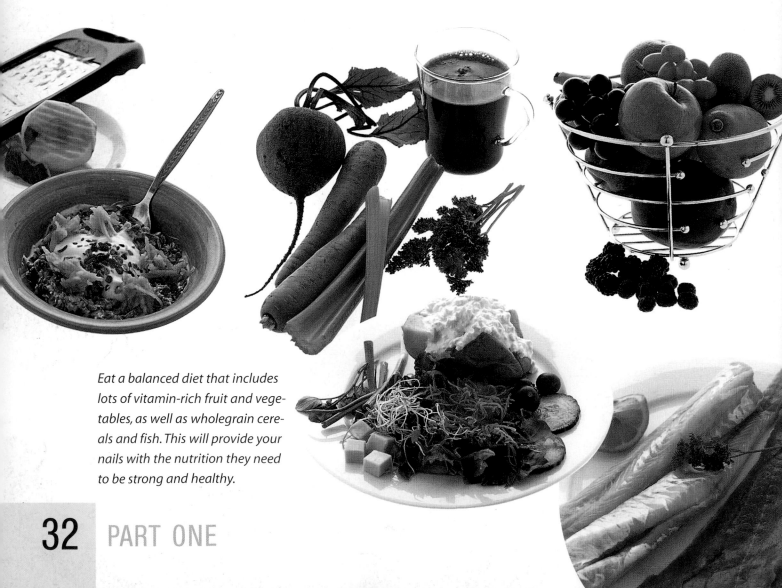

Eat a balanced diet that includes lots of vitamin-rich fruit and vegetables, as well as wholegrain cereals and fish. This will provide your nails with the nutrition they need to be strong and healthy.

Caring for long nails

While long nails and nail art are not always sensible or attractive, everyone has different tastes and lifestyles, and long nails and nail adornment may well fit into yours.

If you choose to have long nails, learn how to use your fingers; get into the habit of using them as if you have just applied a fresh coat of nail polish. Remember that the more knocks your nails suffer, the more likely the tips will break. People are often surprised at how easily nails break, yet few realize that the damage began days – even weeks – earlier.

Long nails are, by nature, weaker than 'normally' shaped nails, and therefore require special attention. Pointed nails have very little support, while oval or square-shaped nails are more likely to survive when long.

Several coats of nail hardener will help to minimize chipping and peeling of the nail enamel. The trick is to find something that protects *and* moisturizes. Nail hardeners with nylon fibres can be very effective tools in your maintenance plan, but prolonged use of hardener can make nails too brittle. Change to a protection basecoat instead (for instance, a thickening gel) if nails are thin.

General reminders for long nails

- *Avoid using nail tips to untie knots or loosen shoelaces.*
- *Use the sides of your fingers to open car doors.*
- *Do not dial the telephone with your fingers; use a pen or pencil.*
- *Use your knuckles to press buttons, such as in elevators.*
- *Use a knife or razor to open boxes and packages, not your nails; nails are not designed as screwdrivers, apple corers or hors d'oeuvre utensils.*
- *Use the pads of your fingers rather than your nails while typing.*
- *Always use rubber gloves when handling household cleaners or bleach, which quickly dry out your nails, leaving them brittle.*
- *When putting on tights or pantyhose, keep your index fingers turned under and use the middle portion of the thumb to pull them up. This not only saves your nails, but also increases the life of your pantyhose.*

TIPS FOR NAIL BITERS

Chronic nail biting deforms the nail plate and damages the tissue surrounding it, resulting in unattractive nails, as well as the introduction of bacteria that may cause illness and minor – but permanent – nail deformities. Regular manicures may help you to become more conscientious of your nails and encourage you to stop biting.

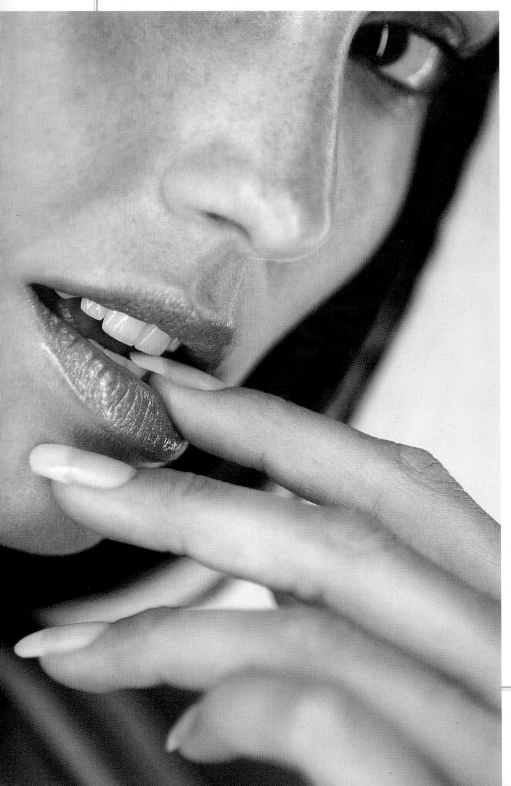

- Devote 10 minutes every day to caring for your nails; as they start to look prettier you will be more inclined to want to stop biting.
- Try using an anti-biting lotion. Once you have stopped for a couple of weeks, your longer nails will provide the incentive to keep up the good work.
- Having short nails does not mean you cannot wear nail varnish; even short nails look better with an application of clear or pale polish.
- Consider wearing false nails or properly applied nail enhancements (see pages 46–47 and 62–70) for a while so your nails have a chance to grow underneath – even the most determined nail biters have trouble gnawing their way through them! A few weeks might be all you need to break the biting habit. However, be aware that nails will be paper thin immediately after artificial nails are removed.
- Carry an emery board with you at all times so you can instantly smooth away straggly edges that tempt you to bite.

COPING WITH FLAKY NAILS

While some women have naturally strong nails, others search endlessly for the solution to stronger nails. Weak, flaky nails are the most common nail complaint. While there is no guaranteed formula that can transform fragile nails into tough talons, here are a few pointers to help you grow more beautiful nails.

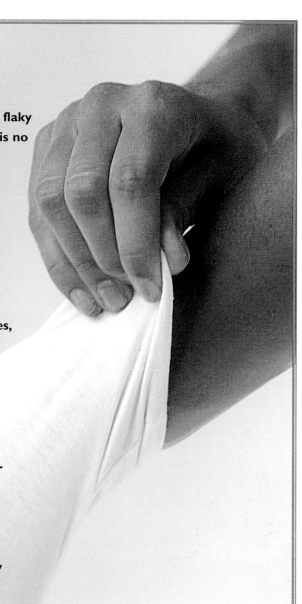

- Always wear rubber gloves when washing up; soaking your nails in water is one sure way to weaken them. Detergents strip the natural oils your nails need for strength. If your hands get too sweaty inside the gloves, wear thin cotton ones underneath to help absorb the moisture and further protect your hands. Also wear gloves for gardening chores to prevent damage.
- Acetone-free nail polish removers are essential as acetone is very drying and serves to further weaken already fragile nails.
- Most reputable nail-care ranges offer a nail strengthener to help prevent splitting and flaking. Apply it underneath your basecoat. Avoid nail strengtheners that contain extremely drying ingredients like formaldehyde, which temporarily toughens the nail but also make it more brittle. Formaldehyde goes by other names in ingredient lists, so watch out for words such as toluene, toluene sulphonamide and toluene sulphonic acid.
- Avoid using your nails as tools; even the toughest nails will not take kindly to being used as screwdrivers, scrapers and levers.
- Get into the habit of applying hand cream each time you have washed your hands to help boost moisture levels and minimize brittle and dry nails.
- Keep your nails short; sensible lengths are less likely to break. Short nails are not only in fahion, but are more practical and attractive.

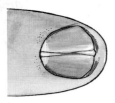

BRITTLE/SPLIT NAIL

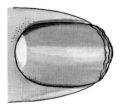

HANGNAIL

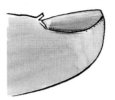

THIN NAIL

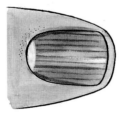

VERTICAL RIDGES

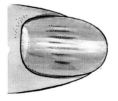

FURROWS

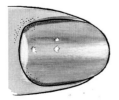

WHITE SPOTS

Nail problems and remedies

Your nails can change texture, colour, thickness or shape – changes that often reflect your inner health. Monitor changes carefully and get appropriate help.

Brittle nails

Onychorrhexis refers to split or brittle nails that are often ridged lengthwise. The condition is caused by injury to the fingers, and abuse of the nails through overexposure to chemical solvents, water, rough handling and drying polish removers. Wear gloves, avoid rough handling and tough detergents, and try using a conditioning treatment.

Hangnails

These are small tears or splits in the cuticle and surrounding tissue. Usually the result of nail biting, they may also be caused by dry skin or injury. If untreated, they may tear and become raw, painful, and subject to infection. Trim with nippers or nail scissors and treat with an antiseptic if the affected area is small.

Thin nails

Like good skin and thick hair, strong nails are a hereditary trait, but vitamin A can help to firm thin nails. Regular grooming and brushing on a nail-strengthening formula may help prevent breakage. As clippers can bend and break your nails, it is a better idea to use scissors for trimming if you really are too rushed to file them with an emery board.

Vertical ridges

Not uncommon in adults, vertical ridges become more widespread as we get older due to a decline in the natural oil and moisture levels in the nail plate. Disruptions in nail growth patterns as a result of illness and nutritional deficiencies also cause ridges. Treat them with regular applications of nourishing nail and cuticle oil.

Furrows

These are corrugations or long ridges that run in either direction across the nail. Ridges across the nail can be caused by high fever, pregnancy or zinc deficiency, while lengthwise corrugations may be triggered by psoriasis (*see* p 39) or poor circulation. Try increasing your zinc intake. Gently buff to smooth out irregularities or fill with ridge-filler and cover with the varnish of your choice.

White spots

White spots on the nail plate (leukonychia) are caused by tiny air bubbles trapped in the nail plate, usually as a result of mild trauma to the nail bed or matrix. Zinc and calcium may help but the spots will gradually grow out. If they bother you, apply varnish to conceal them.

Nail diseases and disorders

Nail infections and diseases can be caused by a number of different conditions. If you have a badly infected nail, see a dermatologist.

Fungal or yeast infections

These can invade the superficial layers of the skin, resulting in infection. Usually germinating their spores alongside the edges of finger- and toenails, some fungal infections caused by microscopic plants invade through a tear in the nail fold. These are normally white or yellowish in colour and affect the texture and shape of the nail as the fungus eats away at the keratin protein of the nail plate. As the infection develops, the nail may darken and discolour, becoming thickened and crumbly.

The first step to treating the problem effectively is to have it diagnosed correctly.

Poor hygiene can cause fungus to develop. Sterilize the tools in your nail kit using an antibacterial spray and never go to a salon that does not sterilize implements after every client.

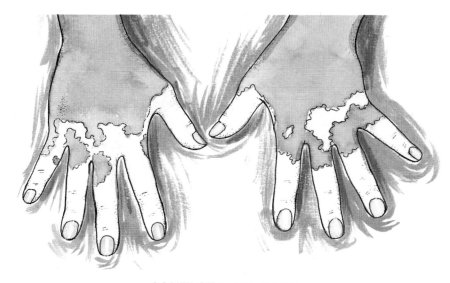

CONTACT DERMATITIS

If a fungus problem persists, consult a dermatologist. Finally, try to avoid biting your nails as this will increase your risk of infection.

Contact dermatitis

This is an allergic reaction to certain substances touching your skin. Symptoms are itching, redness and dryness. When it affects nails and surrounding skin, it is probably caused by irritants such as adhesives, monomers or primers used to secure acrylic nails. Stop using the irritating substance or consult a dermatologist if you are not sure of the cause.

The condition may be confused with psoriasis (*see* page 39) or onychomycosis, which is an infectious disease caused by fungus, resulting in white patches that can be scraped off the nail, or yellowish streaks within the nail.

Deformed nail plate

A nail plate that is shaped like a spoon and is white or opaque is often caused by age, but can also provide clues to common medical problems such as eczema, tumours, anaemia, or chronic infection. The index, ring and middle fingers are most affected. Treat infected nails gently, as the nail plate will be fragile.

Haematoma

Haematoma (or bruised nails) is a condition in which a clot of blood forms between the nail plate and

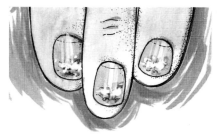

FUNGAL/YEAST INFECTION

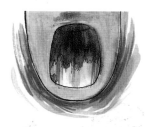

HAEMATOMA

the nail bed. It varies in colour from a dark red to black, and in some cases the nail plate will separate and become infected. New growth will depend on the extent of the damage.

It is usually caused by trauma from impact, such as being hit on the nail with a hammer or, as is common in runners, friction from ill-fitting shoes. Relieve pressure by puncturing the nail with a heated needle to prevent nail loss.

Koilonychia

Commonly known as spoon nails, this is usually caused by an iron deficiency. The nails appear thin and concave, and can exhibit raised ridges. Sudden changes in nail shape may point to internal health problems; consult your GP.

Melanonychia

This is usually associated with vertical pigmented brown or black stripes, or nail 'moles', that form in the nail matrix. This sudden change in the nail plate could indicate a malignant melanoma or lesion that requires medical advice. That said, dark streaks are a fairly frequent and normal occurrence in dark-skinned people.

Onychatrophia

This is also known as atrophy, or wasting away of the nail plate. The nail loses its shine, shrinks and sometimes even falls off. The problem can be caused by injury

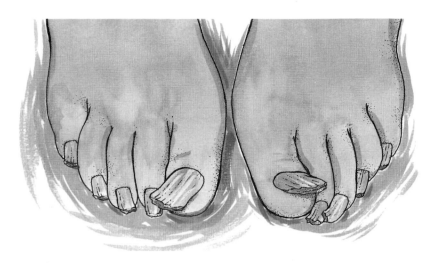

ONYCHOGRYPHOSIS

or internal disease, as well as nutritional or hereditary factors.

Handle this condition carefully. File the nail with a fine emery board and avoid using metal pushers, aggressive detergents and soaps. New nails may grow back once any disease is cured.

Onychauxis

Onychauxis, or hypertrophy, is the overgrowth of nails – a thickening and curving of the nail plate. It is usually caused by internal imbalances, local infection and in some case hereditary factors. File and buff the nail smooth.

Onychogryphosis

This is a condition where the nail plate becomes thick and claw-like, curving inward and sometimes extending over the tip of the finger. Often caused by trauma, it pinches the nail bed painfully. You may need surgery to ease the pain.

Paronychia

Also called a whitlow, this chronic infection of the tissue surrounding the nail results in redness, inflammation and tenderness. Caused by a bacterial or yeast infection, it can occur at the base of the nail, around the whole nail or on the tips of the fingers.

You will be more prone to this problem if you pull your hangnails, suck your thumb or bite

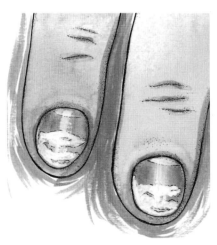

PARONYCHIA

your nails. Having your hands in water for extended periods also increases your risk, so wear gloves and get medical advice on the appropriate treatment.

Pseudomonas

This bacterial infection occurs between the natural nail plate and nail bed. In some cases it occurs between an artificial nail coating and the natural nail plate, especially if worn for extended periods without allowing the natural nail to breathe. It thrives in moist dark places, feeding off dead tissue and bacteria in the nail plate.

Usually, the darker the discoloration, the further into the nail layers the bacteria have travelled. Once treated, it will take several months for the stain to grow out.

Always dry your hands thoroughly as any additional moisture levels allow these bacteria to flourish. Try applying one drop of tea tree oil on the affected area or

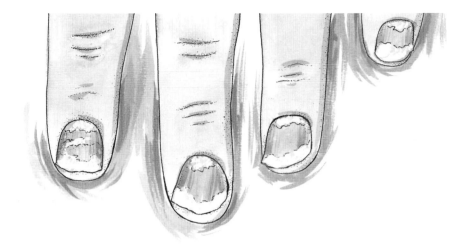

PSORIASIS

soak in a 5 per cent solution several times a day for a few days. An infected nail needs to be analyzed; depending on the cause, an antifungal or antibacterial remedy might need to be applied. If severe, consult a dermatologist.

Psoriasis

This skin condition is characterized by round, reddish dry spots and patches covered with silvery scales. When it affects the nail plate, the nail becomes pitted and dry and may change colour and separate from the nail bed. If severe, the nail plate may disintegrate completely. If psoriasis affects your nails, consult a dermatologist for treatment.

Pterygium

This common condition describes the abnormal growth of the cuticle over the nail plate. It is usually caused by trauma to the matrix

and may even result in the loss of the nail. Never try to remove the pterygium yourself; rather consult a doctor for advice and treatment.

Separation from the nail bed

When the nail separates from the nail bed, the cause may be trauma or a thyroid disorder, but most often the origin is unknown. Carefully trim away the separated nail and seek medical advice.

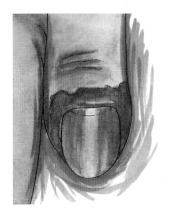

PSEUDOMONAS

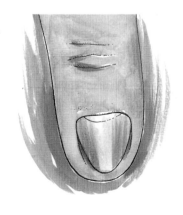

SEPARATION FROM NAIL BED

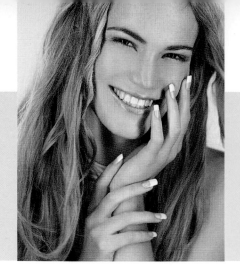

The ultimate manicure

If you are serious in your quest for beautiful nails, you need the right tools for the job. While nothing beats the indulgence of having your nails done professionally, you can also give yourself a manicure at home. All you need are the right tools and the know-how you will find in this chapter.

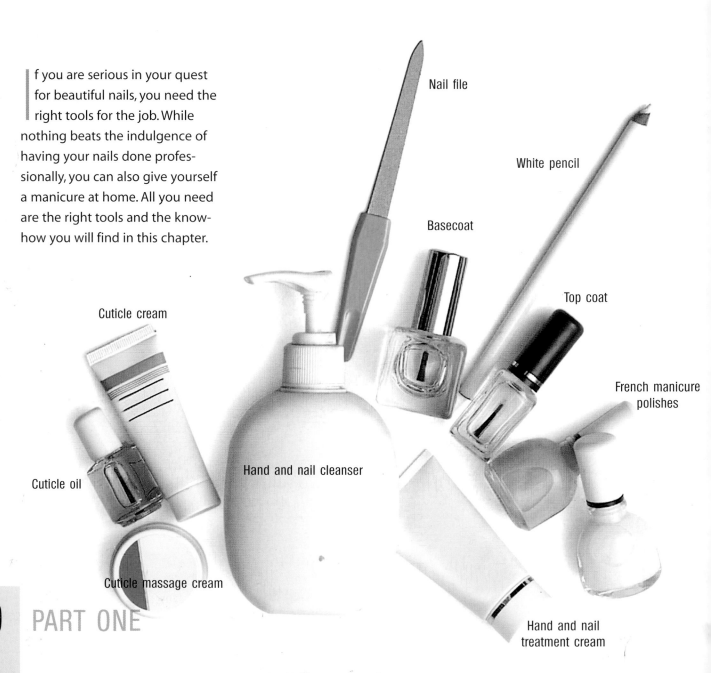

Nail file

White pencil

Basecoat

Top coat

Cuticle cream

French manicure polishes

Cuticle oil

Hand and nail cleanser

Cuticle massage cream

Hand and nail treatment cream

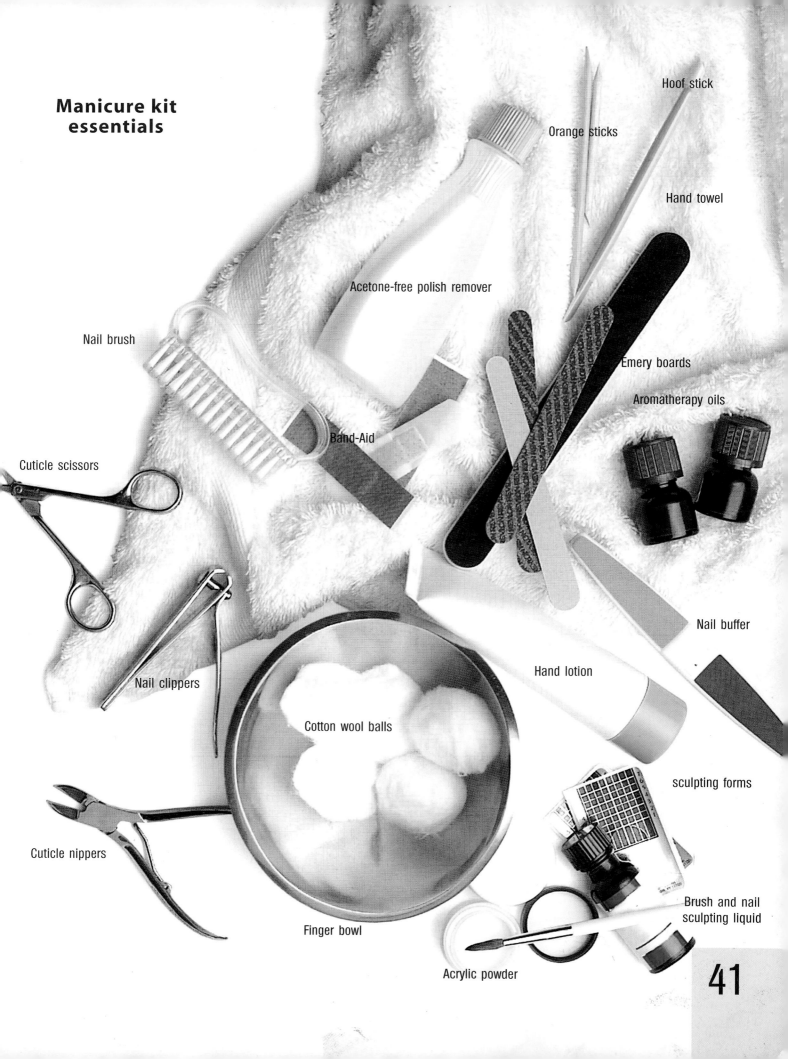

Manicure kit essentials

Hoof stick

Orange sticks

Hand towel

Acetone-free polish remover

Nail brush

Emery boards

Aromatherapy oils

Band-Aid

Cuticle scissors

Nail buffer

Hand lotion

Nail clippers

sculpting forms

Cotton wool balls

Cuticle nippers

Brush and nail
sculpting liquid

Finger bowl

Acrylic powder

41

Manicure kit essentials

Acetone-free polish remover: to remove nail polish before the manicure begins. Avoid acetone or its chemical relatives, which damage the surface of the nail, affecting the lustre, and weakening and thinning the nail plate.

Aromatherapy oils: for a relaxing mood or to relieve stress.

Cotton balls: for removing nail polish, and for wrapping orange sticks to push back your cuticles. Cotton balls are very absorbent and do not leave fibre behind.

Cuticle softeners: these include both cuticle cream and cuticle oil. Softening cuticles makes them easier to push back. Softeners also loosen stubborn skin stuck to the nail bed. They come in formulations from clear liquids you paint on to thick creams you massage into the cuticle. Avoid products containing potassium hydroxice, which can damage nails.
a. Cuticle cream: smoothing a specially blended cream around the cuticle area softens the surrounds and prevents hangnails from developing. These usually contain fats and waxes, such as lanolin, cocoa butter, petroleum jelly and beeswax.
b. Cuticle oil: vitamin E-enriched oils and sweet almond oil, applied regularly, will condition the cut-

icle area and maintain it at optimum health. Cuticle oils may also contain mineral oil, jojoba oil and palm nut oil.

Emery boards: a coarsely grained, double-sided one is best to shorten or smooth nails, a fine-grained version for final smoothing.

Finger bowl: for soaking fingernails; fill it with warm, soapy water.

Hand lotion: to promote supple skin by hydrating and helping to seal moisture into the skin.

Hand towel: for drying your hands, and to place under your hands as you apply nail polish.

Hoof stick: a manicure stick with a rubber tip shaped like a hoof, used to push back your cuticles.

Nailbrush: use a nailbrush in the morning and evening for cleaning hands, nails and cuticles. Replace it when bristles lose their density.

Nail buffer: these come in all shapes and sizes, usually combining three buffing surfaces that help to smooth any ridges from nail surfaces, as well as to add sheen. Used gently in a swift back-and-forth manner, they will smooth, shine and buff the nails to give an excellent finish.

Nail cleansers: usually a liquid soap that is added to the water in the finger bowl.

Nail scissors: more gentle on the nails, scissors are often preferred to clippers for ultimate precision.

Nipper: this is a useful tool for trimming hangnails and should feature a pointed tip to allow a precise trim.

Orange stick: use an orange stick (traditionally made of orangewood) wrapped in cottonwool to push back cuticles. It can be used instead of the nailbrush to clean under the nail.

Clear basecoat: to provide a foundation for the nail polish.

Clear or tinted nail polish: the main coat of polish in the colour of your choice; a clear polish will last longer without showing chips or peels.

Topcoat: a protective and durable coating for the polish. It lengthens the lifespan of coloured polish because it helps to prevent chipping.

White pencil: gently drawing the pencil under damp nails will help to simulate the attractive look of a French manicure.

Step-by-step manicure

Looking after your hardworking nails can be a relaxing experience. Allow time for a manicure every 7–14 days, with weekly time for touch-ups. When performed correctly, a manicure will protect your nails and help improve your image. If a DIY manicure is not for you, look at the pointers for what you can expect at a salon (*see* pages 74–75). However, with practice, it is not difficult to achieve an expert, professional-looking manicure. Follow these steps methodically and meticulously to create good-looking, immaculate nails. And remember, a man's manicure is exactly the same, except for the application of nail polish.

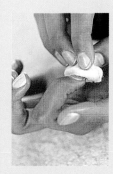 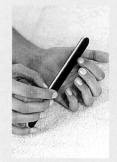

1 Remove all traces of old enamel by moistening some cottonwool with the remover of your choice. Press it onto the nail and hold for a few seconds, then swipe it toward the free edge. Change cottonwool often, as the remover cannot perform well if it is saturated with old enamel. Dark-pigmented enamels are hardest to remove, and the old polish may get on your skin or underneath the free edge. If this happens, wrap a small piece of cottonwool on the end of an orange stick, saturate it with remover, and clean the enamel from the cuticle line and under the free edge of the nail.

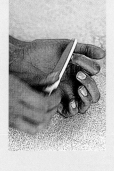

2 Use a coarse-grade emery board to remove length or perfect the free edge or tip by filing from the outside corner to the centre of the nail. Never saw back and forth across the tip; this can disrupt the nail-plate layers and cause splitting and peeling. The ideal shape of the free edge should mirror the shape of the cuticle, i.e. oval cuticle = oval free edge.

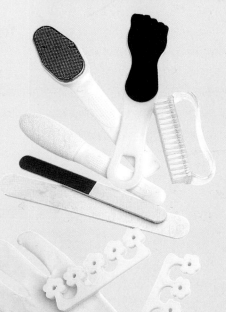

3 To seal the tip, use the three-way buffer: the black part to refine, the white part to semi-shine and the grey part to finish. This will seal the layers of the free edge in order to further prevent any splitting or peeling.

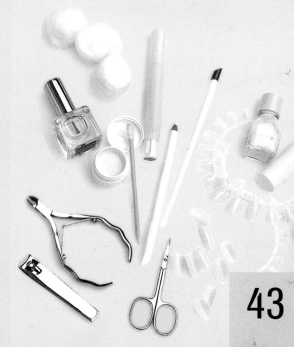

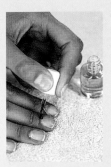

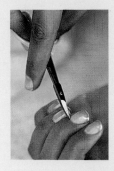

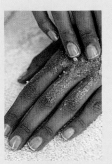

4 Apply cuticle softener (cream, oil or lotion) all around the cuticle area. Then immerse your nails in the soaking dish for no more than three minutes; soaking for longer will fully saturate the nail plate, causing it to swell.

6 Holding the cuticle nippers/ scissors in one hand, nip or clip any loose tags of skin you were unable to remove with the cuticle pusher. *Never* cut live skin; be very careful to trim only the dead tissue. If no translucent tissue has been pushed from the nail plate, or there are no tags of dead skin, there is no need to trim anything.

8 At this point, you may wish to exfoliate your hands by dispensing a small amount of sloughing lotion into the palm of one hand. Distribute it evenly between your palms, then massage into the palms of the hand and fingers, being especially gentle with the back of the hands. Massage for just a few minutes, then rinse or wipe clean with a wet towel and dry thoroughly.

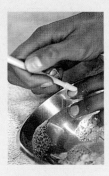

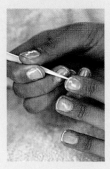

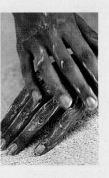

5 Remove the fingers from the soaking dish. Holding the orange stick or metal cuticle pusher much as you would a pencil, push the cuticle skin from the nail-plate surface back toward the live tissue. Do not use downward force, which could cause damage to the nail matrix.

7 Using the orange stick or the curved end of the metal cuticle pusher, clean under the free edge of the nail, but be careful – any tear or break in the seal between the nail plate and the nail bed is the perfect entry point for bacterial micro-organisms that may cause an infection.

9 Apply moisturizing lotion, and massage it into the skin until it is completely absorbed.

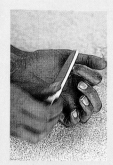

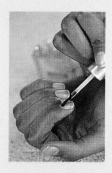

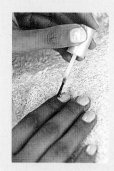

10   Do not file the nail plate as this may cause splitting and cracking. You may buff at this stage to get a natural shine, but do not file ridges to smooth them. Rather use a ridge filler to smooth out the nails. To buff, use the three-way buffer; using the three sides in turn creates a high-gloss shine and helps to seal the nail-plate surface from staining and dehydration by 'plasticizing' the surface layer.

12   Begin your polish application with one thin basecoat. *Always* use a basecoat, which is designed to adhere to the nail plate to pro-tect and seal the surface and bond with the coloured polish. Choose a basecoat suitable for your nail type – for example, a nail hardener for weak nails or a ridge filler for uneven nails.

14   Finish with a thin application of topcoat to seal the surface. The inherent hardness of the topcoat will help to keep the polish fresh for a little longer.

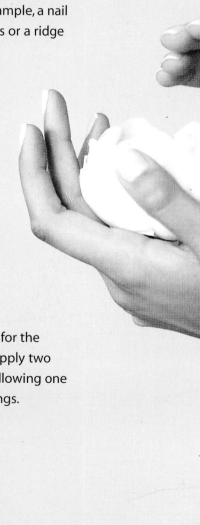

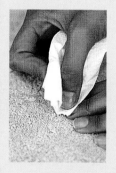

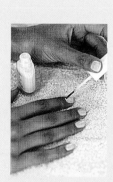

11   Wash, rinse and dry your hands and nails to remove all sur-face traces of nail filings, lotions or oils. If your skin and nails are excessively oily and you have used any type of oil, lotion or cream during your manicure process, you may wish to swipe the nail plate with a dampened pad to be sure all traces have been removed. Enamel will not adhere success-fully to an oily surface.

13   Allow one minute for the basecoat to dry, then apply two thin coats of enamel, allowing one minute between coatings.

Faking it

False nails offer the ideal solution for women who battle to grow their own. There are now several techniques to make up for chewed or unsightly nails. The term 'artificial nail enhancement' includes any process that lengthens, thickens or otherwise alters the appearance of the natural nail by artificial means. These include the application of tips, acrylic liquid and powder systems, gel systems, sculpting on a form, any type of fabric wrap or even the application of a full preformed artificial nail.

Be aware that acrylic nails contain chemicals that can cause allergic reactions, damage nails and encourage fungal infections that may turn the bed of the nail green if used incorrectly. Acrylic nails prevent nail ventilation, allowing fungi and bacteria to grow (*see* pseudomonas, page 39). There is also some evidence that ingredients in acrylic nails can penetrate the nail's matrix.

Infection is not the only potential problem if you keep your nails permanently under wraps. Others are cracking, splitting and discoloration. If you decide that false nails are for you, take note of these nail-saving tactics:

- Avoid wearing false nails for more than a week at a time, and give your own nails at least two days' break in-between.

- If you notice any green or yellowish discoloration of the nail bed, consult your doctor or dermatologist; it could signify a fungal or bacterial infection.
- Be careful when cleaning under your nails; use a brush and soapy water or an ear-bud, never an orange stick, which can be quite sharp, unless covered with a twist of cottonwool.
- Replenish lost moisture by giving nails an oil massage.

Acrylic nails: To create acrylic nails, a nail technician mixes together two ingredients called powdered polymer and liquid monomer. When combined, the powder and liquid react to form a plastic-like paste. This is smoothed onto the nail, where it hardens. Note that the monomer used in acrylics is potentially irritating to sensitive skins.

Acrylic tips: Tips do not cover the entire nail but are attached mid-way up the natural nail, and the surface is later buffed down to hide the join (*see* page 70). Acrylic is then placed over the entire nail and tip.

Built-up tips: Oval paper or metal is inserted under the nail before acrylic is painted on and allowed to set. Finally, the tip is filed to your chosen shape.

Gel nails: These are created by applying layers of acrylic gel to the nail; the layers combine and harden to form a solid natural-looking nail enhancement. (*See* the DIY instructions on pages 64–70.)

False nails: These can be applied professionally in a salon or you can apply them at home, using an inexpensive nail enhancement kit. They come with their own adhesive and can be cut and filed to a shape and size that suits you.

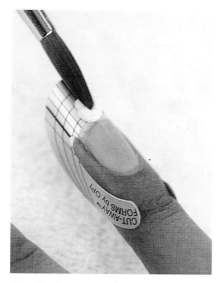
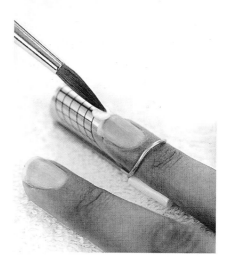

Acrylic tips are sculpted on a form. Various types of guides can be used.

Stick-on nails: Pre-cast plastic nail shapes are applied with a special fixative or double-sided tape. They can be applied at home and look natural as long as you choose the right size. Most suppliers offer a variety of nail widths.

Patching: If you split or break a nail, it can be repaired with a patch that works on the same principle as a sticking plaster on skin. Inexpensive DIY repair-a-nail kits are available for you to use at home, or patches can be applied at a salon by a professional.

Wraps: To add a stronger layer to the nail to help nails grow longer without breaking or splitting, nail wraps use sheets of fibreglass, linen, or silk. To create nail wraps, a nail technician takes small pieces of fabric mesh and sticks them to your nails with an adhesive. After buffing the surface to smooth it, a sealant is applied to keep out moisture and discourage the wrap from lifting. Wraps can also be used to rescue a single broken nail. (*See* also the DIY instructions on pages 64–65.)

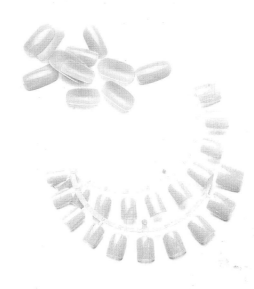

Try stick-on nails for an instant lift: to look natural choose the right size.

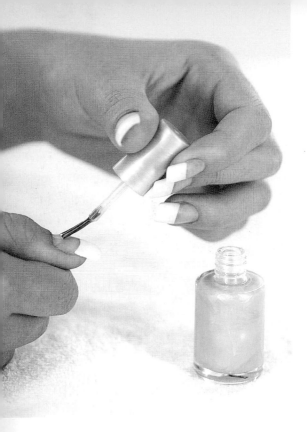

Nail varnish

Manicured nails can be traced back some 4000 years to southern Babylon, where noblemen used solid gold implements to manicure their fingernails and toenails. But nail decoration goes back even further to 6000 years ago, when the Egyptians were decorating their nails by buffing them with henna, the deepest red indicating the highest status.

It is generally believed that the Chinese invented nail enamel some 5000 years ago, and the desire for very long nails first began during China's Ming dynasty (1368-1644). At this time, aristocratic women started to grow their nails up to 25cm (10in) long as a sign that they performed no manual labour. To protect their nails, they frequently sheathed them in gold or silver. Chinese men also grew long nails as a sign of their masculinity and to protect themselves from evil.

It is also known that the Romans were applying 'fingernail polish' made of animal fat and blood around AD100.

Today, our fascination with long, beautiful nails continues to grow, and has been responsible for establishing a multibillion-dollar industry. Read on to find out everything you need to know about nail varnish.

Basecoat

Basecoat serves many purposes, including priming, giving protection and adding strength. Choosing a basecoat can be confusing, as many variations are available. Just remember that basecoat needs a clean, oil-free surface to adhere to, otherwise it will probably peel off almost as soon as it dries.

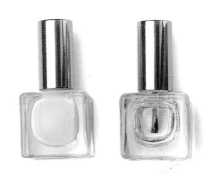

Basecoat and nail strengthener are essential to your nail care regimen.

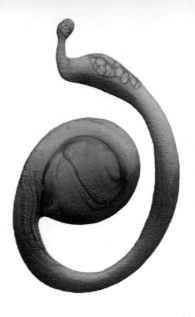

Antifungal basecoat

Standard basecoats are primers that provide some strength, but their primary function is to assist nail varnish to glide on smoothly and to help to prevent darker shades from staining your nails.

When a basecoat contains added ingredients for strength it is known as *nail strengthener*.

Ridge fillers are basecoats containing silk, talc or other particles to help fill in depressions. If your nails are ridged or peeling at the tip, ridge fillers can ensure a smooth finish.

Antifungal basecoats are formulated with ingredients that will help to kill micro-organisms that cause infection.

Nail fortifiers or nail-growth formulas are growth formulas consisting of clear varnish infused with epoxy or formaldehyde resins and polyvinyl butyral. Some contain calcium. Nail fortifiers can be worn under or over your nail varnish, or worn alone.

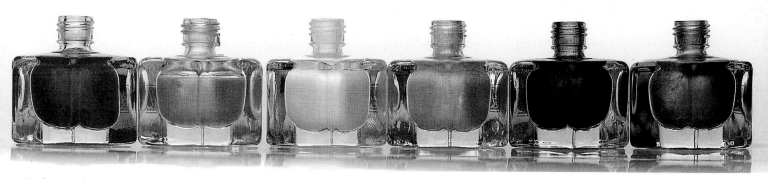

Nail varnishes come in an astonishing array of shades and types – from plain to pearlized and metallic.

Topcoat

Topcoats are clear polish designed to protect your manicure from chipping, flaking and peeling. They are similar to basecoats but dry more quickly and usually feature a glossier finish.

Many nail technicians and manicurists suggest painting on a fresh layer of topcoat every day to extend the life of your manicure.

The perfect polish

Most people want beautiful nails, and whether they are short or long, a beautifully applied coating of coloured enamel is the finishing touch to your manicure.

To begin with, always be sure your polish is fresh. Enamel that has been allowed to thicken will not apply thinly or evenly, will tend to bubble or streak, and will not adhere properly.

Polish thickens because it is volatile – that is, the solvents that keep it in a fluid state evaporate quickly when exposed to air. If a bottle remains open during application, or if it is exposed to heat, the solvents evaporate and the enamel becomes thick, gooey, and stringy. Store polish in a cool, dark place away from heat and keep the neck of the bottle clean to prevent it from thickening.

Begin your application by turning the bottle upside down then rolling it between the palms of your hands (*see* below). Avoid shaking the bottle as this creates bubbles of air in the enamel, which might transfer to the finished surface after application.

The perfect polish is applied by first stroking a basecoat down the centre of the nail plate from cuticle to free edge, then stroking each side in turn. Three to four strokes on each nail are sufficient to distribute the varnish evenly. Additional stroking will only lift and move the enamel, leaving behind streaks and/or bare spots on the nail surface. Leave a tiny margin all around the cuticle and sides of each nail to ensure that the polish does not touch your skin and that it adheres properly to the nail plate.

Remember that oil is a separating medium and your skin contains oils and moisture, so it is best to remove all traces of oil with nail varnish remover before you start.

Apply the coloured enamel in the same manner, allowing enough time for each coat to dry. Apply a thin layer each time. If the pigments in the enamel are not even after the second coating, allow an extra minute before applying a third coat. The pigments in some red or metallic enamels tend to separate during application and may require a third coating for even colour distribution. Allow one to three minutes after the third coat before applying your topcoat or sealer.

Nail enamel dries from the first coat up to the last, and the solvents in the enamel must evaporate before the coatings become hardened. Pausing as long as you can between coatings will produce a smoother, more brilliant surface. If you apply coatings that are too thick or too close together, or you use enamel that has thickened with time, it will smudge, dent or peel from the nail entirely. Remember, applying the coatings too quickly is the main reason for uneven texture, and is especially pronounced in high temperatures and humidity.

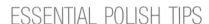

ESSENTIAL POLISH TIPS

- **Allow your nail varnish to dry slowly. Waiting for polish to dry can be tiresome, but the more slowly it dries, the better the finish. Forcing it to dry quickly by using heat or chemical dryers results in excessive shrinkage and cracking; heat causes the polish to expand and lift away from the nail. Formulations that use rapidly evaporating solvents tend to bubble and pit more, or produce uneven surfaces. Blowing on the polish will lower adhesion and gloss, so be patient.**
- **Do not count on glitter polish to stay on. The glitter itself does not adhere to nails, so tends to chip more quickly than conventional colours.**
- **Use a one-coat polish and a fast-drying topcoat only if you are in a rush. Otherwise, stick to regular formulations as they last longer, and to standard topcoats, which are shinier and give greater protection.**

Broken nail emergencies

The first thing to do with a broken nail is to secure it to prevent further damage until you can get home or to a nail salon.

If the nail is torn but not completely broken off, try wrapping the fingertip with tape or plaster – first up and over the tip and then around the nail. Make sure you keep a bit of slack inside so the nail is not bent. Band-Aids especially designed for fingertips work best. If you use tape, first protect the nail surface with a bit of tissue so the tape will not stick to the nail. An added benefit of covering the fingertip is that you will naturally avoid using that finger, thus minimizing further damage.

Once you get home, use a small pair of scissors to gently cut away the tape. Now you can assess the damage. Do not pick at the nail. If it is just a slight tear on the side, you may get by simply with using extra coats of a nail strengthener containing nylon fibres. It may also be a good idea to shorten the nail slightly so it will be less likely to bang into things, which would cause more damage.

If the nail is completely off, or torn more than one-quarter of the width of the nail, you need to take more serious measures. Keep an emergency nail repair kit on hand that contains both powdered and liquid acrylic, as well as a circular nail buffer.

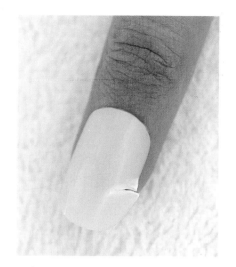 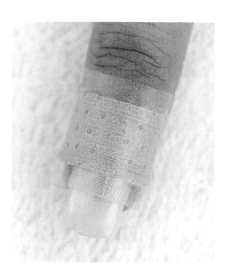

When you tear a nail, tape it with plaster to preserve it until you can fix it.

1. Clean the nail with soap, then rinse it with water and allow it to dry completely.
2. Apply the acrylic, according to directions, in a thick coat that covers the entire nail. Let this dry *completely*, then very carefully buff the nail down to a smooth surface that forms a 'cap' over the broken nail. Keep the nail as short as possible; the longer the nail, the more likely you will bang and break it.
3. Apply a second coat and buff it down again. Some kits come with a thin silk or nylon sheet to be placed between the coats for added strength. Take your time to create a realistic cap over the nail.
4. Once dried, make sure you apply a coat of hardener with nylon fibres daily. When the natural nail has grown long enough, remove the cap by soaking it in polish remover and prying it off very carefully.

Pry it a bit, then soak, then repeat as often as needed to get it off with the least damage.
5. This is not a perfect method, but works well. Keep in mind that if you constantly remove the polish, you will weaken the cap with the polish remover and probably need to start the process all over again.
6. As the nail grows, the base may look a bit odd as the base of the cap becomes exposed. You may need to remove the polish and touch up the cap a bit on the edges; it is best just to leave it with the cap until it has grown enough to expose the natural nail.
7. Basically, if a nail breaks, accept that it will never be as good as new until it grows back naturally. Of course, the easier approach is to accept the loss and trim the other nails down a bit so it does not look so awkward until it grows back.

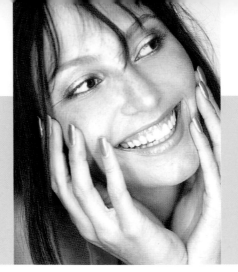

Manicures: step by step

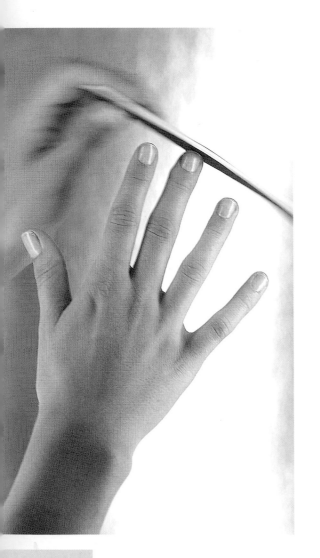

The home manicure

Taking care of your hands should be a regular part of your beauty routine. Try to schedule a home manicure every two or three weeks and allow time in-between for touch-ups. Travelling to a salon, getting a manicure and waiting for your nails to dry can sometimes take too long, so it often makes sense to do it yourself.

1 Partially saturate a cotton ball with varnish remover and work quickly to whisk off old varnish from the base of the nail to the tip. Try not to smear the remover into the cuticle or the surrounding skin. Avoid removers that contain acetone (or any of its chemical relatives), even if they have conditioners. Acetone and its cousins will usually dry out your nails. Quickly rinse off all traces of remover with warm water and dry thoroughly.

2 Shape your nails by filing from one edge of the nail to the centre, and then from the other edge back to the centre. Always hold the emery board at a 45-degree angle so that you are filing mainly the underside of the nail. Repeat on all of your nails. Remember that the most natural and easiest-to-manage shape – not to mention the strongest – is a slightly squared oval. Try to mirror the shape of your nail at the base for the most flattering effect.

3 Dampen your hands and massage them with an exfoliator. You could try a commercial product or a mixture of coarse sea-salt and essential oil to rev up circulation.

4 Soak your fingers in a bowl of lukewarm water.

5 Scrub nails gently with a soft-bristled brush and dry hands thoroughly with a soft towel.

6 Apply cuticle oil or cuticle softener. Massage well into the base of the nails. Leave to work for a few minutes, then gently push cuticles back with a hoof stick or

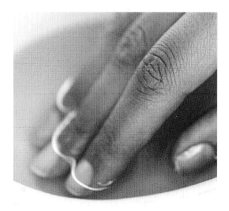

1 **REMOVE OLD VARNISH**

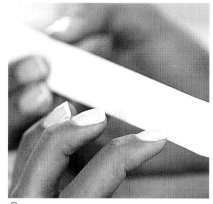

2 **FILE TO SHAPE**

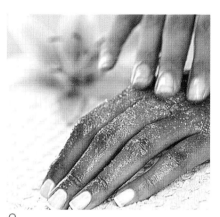

3 **EXFOLIATE**

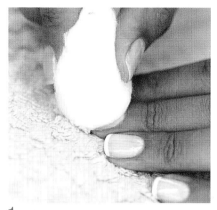

4 **SOAK**

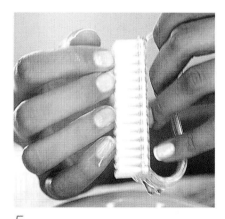

5 **SCRUB**

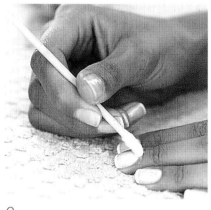

6 **PUSH BACK CUTICLE**

FILING TIPS

- Do not file nails when they are wet; they are more liable to break.

- Do not saw backward and forward, which can cause the nail layers to split and separate.

- File in one direction only, with long, smooth strokes. Use the smooth side of the emery board and never file in the corners.

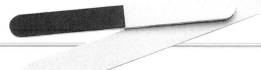

cottonwool-covered orange stick. Wipe off residue with a tissue and rinse nails in warm water to remove all cream/oil.

7 Nip away any ragged excess cuticle or hangnails with a cuticle nipper. Be careful not to cut into the mantle, which can lead to infection.

8 Moisturize cuticles with cuticle oil or moisturizer.

9 Massage with hand cream (*see* pages 78–79 for the right massage technique).

10 Run a white pencil under your nails to brighten them.

11 Remove all signs of cream, then apply nail varnish in three coats: clear basecoat, followed by polish, topped with clear topcoat to lock in colour. Allow the basecoat to dry for three minutes before you start to apply polish. This acts as a foundation for the polish and helps prevent stains. Apply nail polish in two thin coats using three strokes from base to tip: first stroke polish up the centre, then

stroke along each side. Let the first layer of colour dry for three minutes and the second for five minutes. Finally, brush on a topcoat to lock in colour and protect the polish.

For an alternative to nail polish, try nail buffing. It will shine your nails and smooth ridges. For a natural gloss, buff nails gently in one direction, with downward strokes from the base to the free edge. Raise the buffer after each stroke. Do about 10 strokes on each nail.

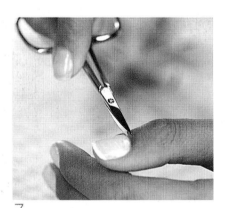
7 **NIP EXCESS CUTICLE**

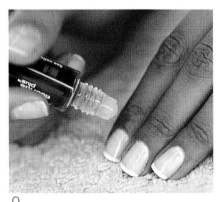
8 **MOISTURIZE CUTICLES**

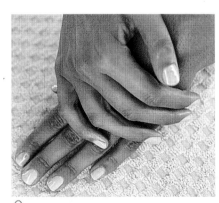
9 **MASSAGE**

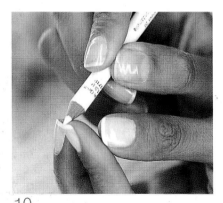
10 **USE WHITE PENCIL**

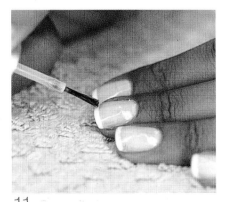
11 **APPLY VARNISH**

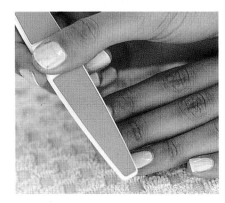
OR BUFF TO SHINE

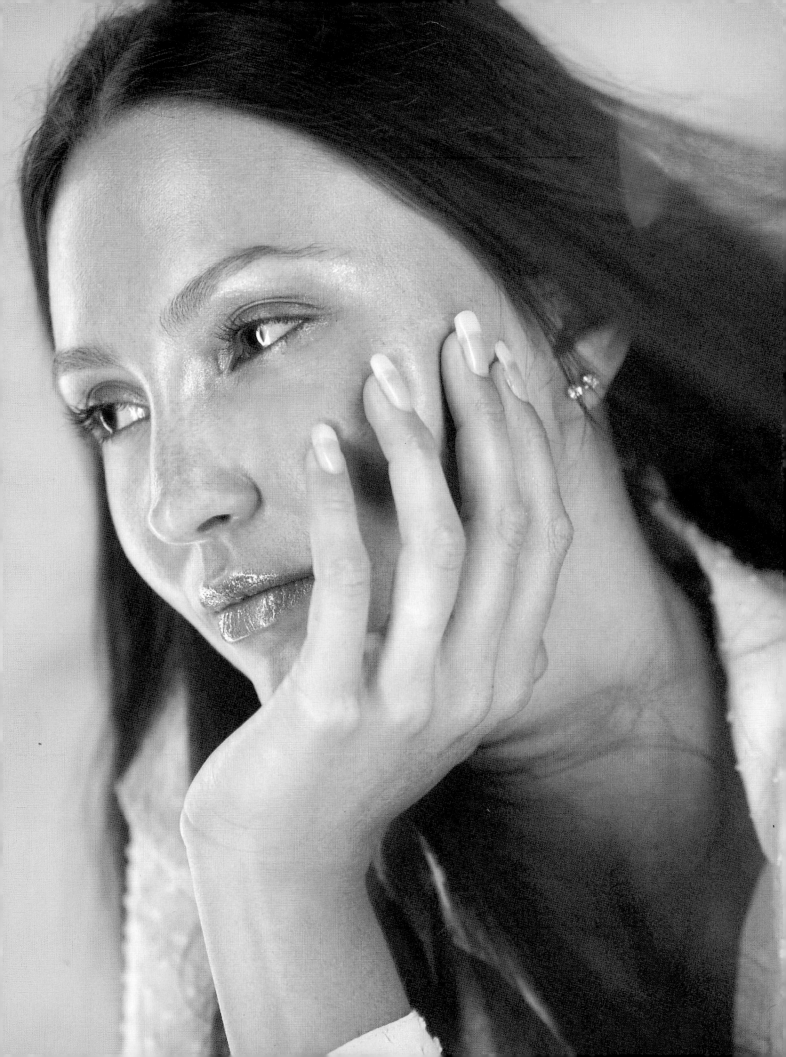

The French manicure

This neutral look makes nails look clean and healthy and suits all occasions. Although it takes a lot of practice, it is worth the effort once you see the finished effect. Most polish ranges include soft pink and white shades that enable you to create an attractive French manicure.

1 Follow the home manicure steps (*see* pages 52–54) through to the filing process, then apply a thin basecoat.

2 Apply white polish to the tip. Start at one side and sweep the loaded brush toward the centre of the nail in a diagonal swipe. Repeat from the other side. This will create a 'V' shape, which you can correct by filling the open top of the 'V'. Repeat on all nails.

3 When dry, apply sheer varnish (beige, clear or pink) over entire nail. Experiment with various colour options in order to create sophisticated variations on the classic French manicure.

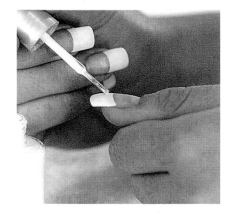

1 **FILE TO SHAPE**

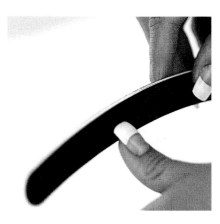

2 **PAINT TIPS WHITE**

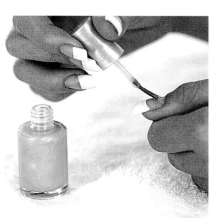

3 **APPLY SHEER COAT**

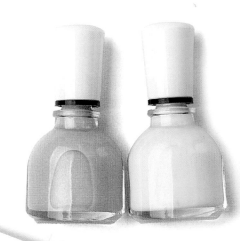

TIPS

- **A simpler option is to find some pre-cut, self-adhesive French manicure guides. Lift the edge of one strip and remove from the backing** paper. **Place it across the nail to divide the tip from the rest of the nail, leaving a small strip. Press down firmly to smooth out any ripples. Repeat on all nails. Apply white nail varnish to the nail** tip and allow to dry. **Remove guides and apply sheer varnish over entire nail.**
- **Another option is to run a white pencil under the free edges of your nails to accentuate the tips.**

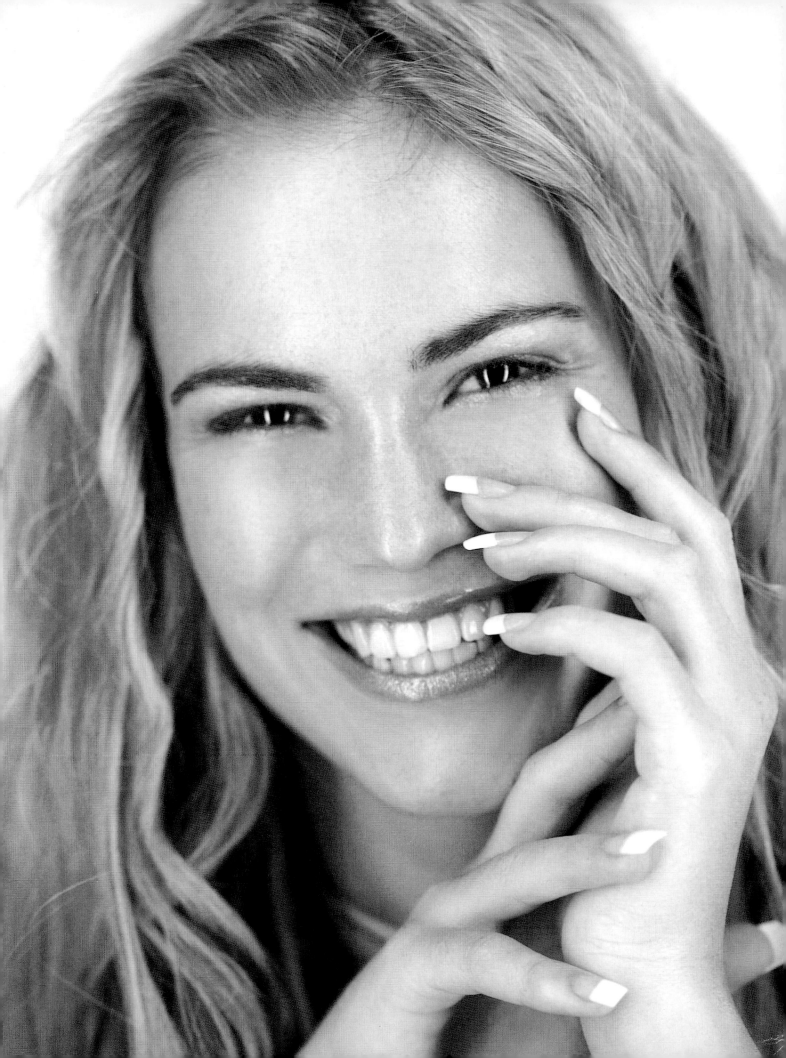

Vamp nails: short and dark

Dark nails, especially short ones, look chic and sophisticated. Remember that dark varnishes can stain your nails so basecoat is essential to protect your nails, especially if you wear dark nails continuously. A steady, practised hand is essential when applying dark nail polish.

1 Follow the basic steps of a home manicure (*see* pages 52–54) to shape and condition your nails, then apply a layer of basecoat to prevent the dark pigment from staining your nails. Allow the clear basecoat to dry for three minutes to ensure that you achieve a solid foundation.

2 Start applying a dark shade of nail varnish on the little finger of your right hand and work inward to avoid smudging. Apply a stripe of polish down the centre of your nail, followed by stripes on either side to finish. The side strokes will meet with and overlap the centre one. To prevent messy application, avoid overloading the brush. Apply two or three thin coats, allowing each to dry completely.

3 Use a nail polish corrector or an orange stick covered with a little cotton wool dipped in nail varnish remover to clean up the sides and the cuticles, as well as underneath the free edge of the nail.

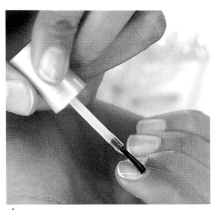

1 **APPLY BASECOAT**

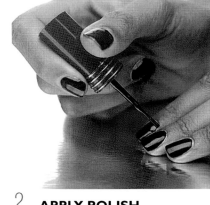

2 **APPLY POLISH**

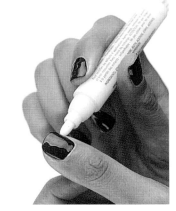

3 **CLEAN CUTICLES**

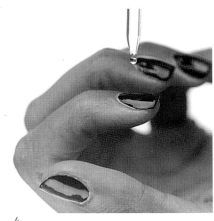

4 **APPLY LIQUID NAIL DRY**

4 Apply topcoat to prevent chipping and add shine. Liquid nail dry can be used to prevent smudging and speed up the drying process, but remember quick-dry solutions usually contain acetone, which can parch your nails.

> TIP
> **Soak stained nails in a solution of a capful of hydrogen peroxide to a cup warm water. Then use a soft brush to scrub each nail.**

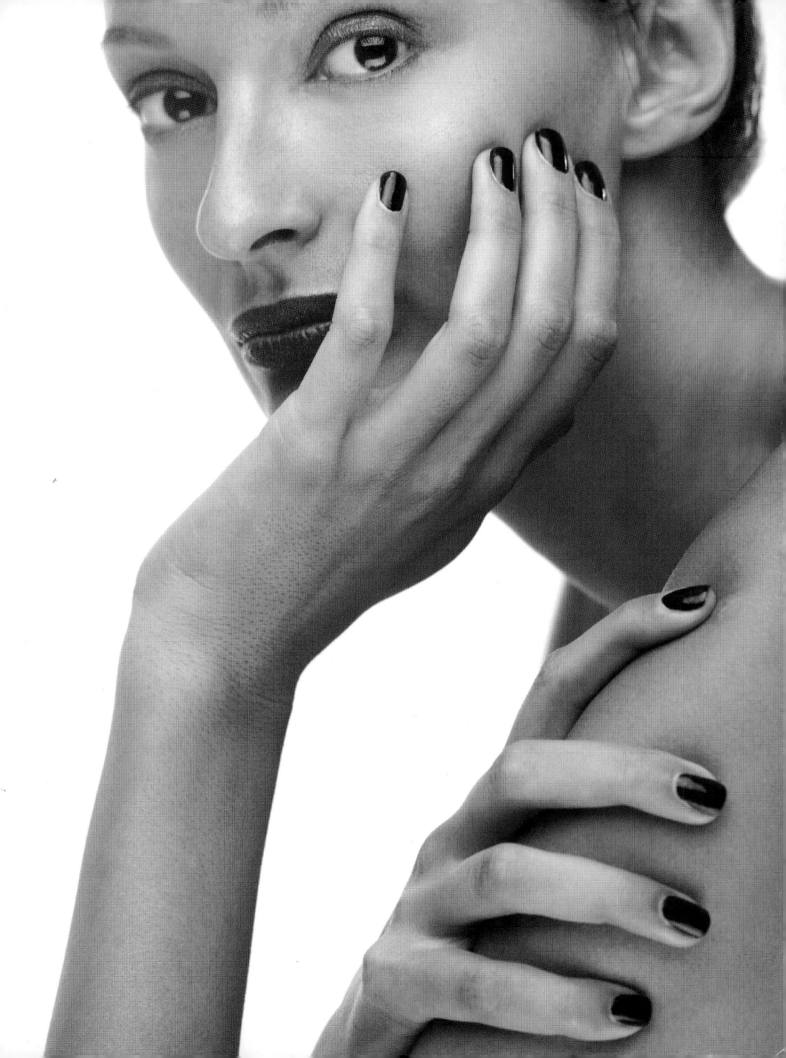

Henna nail paste, or Mehndi

Mehndi is the ancient traditional art of adorning hands, fingers, forearms and toes with non-permanent dye paste made from the leaves of the henna plant. Patterns vary from floral patterns in Arab countries to lacy paisley designs in India. Believed to have healing properties, it is usually used in marriage rites to protect the bride. It is fun to wear but tricky to do, so try this simple, stencilled version instead.

1 Although henna is tradition-ally painted on freehand, this requires an artistic and steady hand. For a simpler version, look for self-adhesive stencils and secure these by pressing firmly into place.

2 In a non-porous bowl, mix up a thick paste of henna pow-der, a teaspoon of coffee gran-ules and some hot water. The resulting paste is a soft green in colour but leaves behind a neutral shade of brown.

3 Spread the paste thickly over the stencil, concentrating on the exposed areas. Leave to dry for as long as possible; the longer you leave it, the more intense the henna stain. Overnight would be ideal.

4 Once the henna paste has dried, peel off the stencil care-fully to reveal the delicate lace pattern beneath. Rinse off any remaining paste and pat your hands dry. You can expect the stain to last for a few days on the skin (though it lasts longer when used on nails).

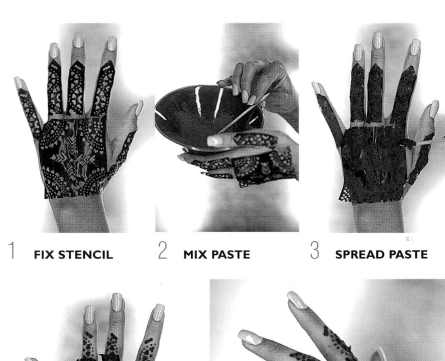

1 FIX STENCIL   2 MIX PASTE   3 SPREAD PASTE

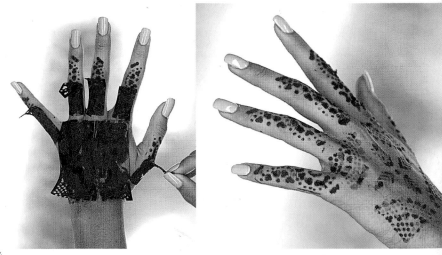

4 PEEL OFF STENCIL   THE FINISHED EFFECT

TIP

Apply a thick blob of henna paste on each clean, dry nail to help strengthen and condition them, but bear in mind that on nails the stain can last from four to six weeks.

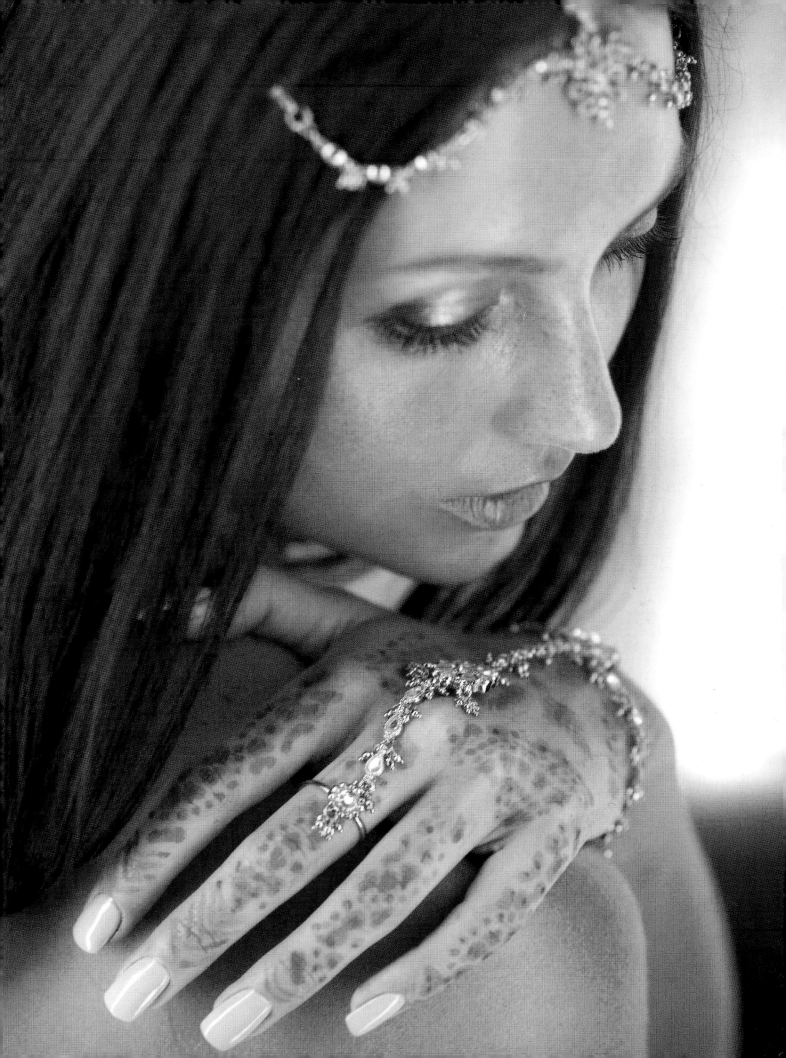

Artificial nails

Artificial nails offer an easy solution for growing out your natural nails, provide instant gratification, can be applied at home, and are ideal for replacing a broken nail. They look natural if you choose the right size, eliminate the white plastic effect and file them into a convincing shape.

1 Clean and dry your natural nails. File and condition them ready to attach artificial nails.

2 Select the correct nail size for each nail. If necessary, file the sides for an exact fit.

3 Spread a thin, even layer of nail glue over your entire nail or over the part of the artificial nail that will be attached to your natural nail.

4 Place the false nail up to – but not touching – the cuticle. Press firmly for a few seconds. File off any rough edges.

5 Apply two coats of nail varnish of your choice and seal with a layer of topcoat.

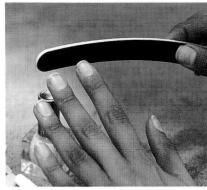

1 **FILE NAILS**

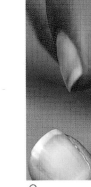

2 **CHECK FIT**

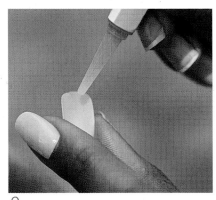

3 **APPLY GLUE**

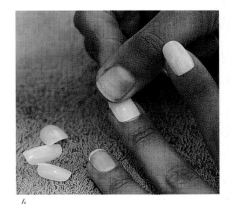

4 **PLACE ON BARE NAIL**

TIPS

- **Use non-acetone polish remover to remove artificial nails, soaking until they dissolve. Never break or peel them off as this damages your natural nail.**

- **Do not wear artificial nails for longer than a few weeks at a time; your natural nails need a breather.**

- **Never use household glue; use special nail adhesives.**

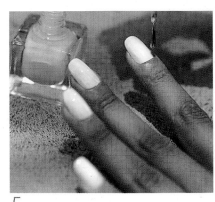

5 **APPLY VARNISH**

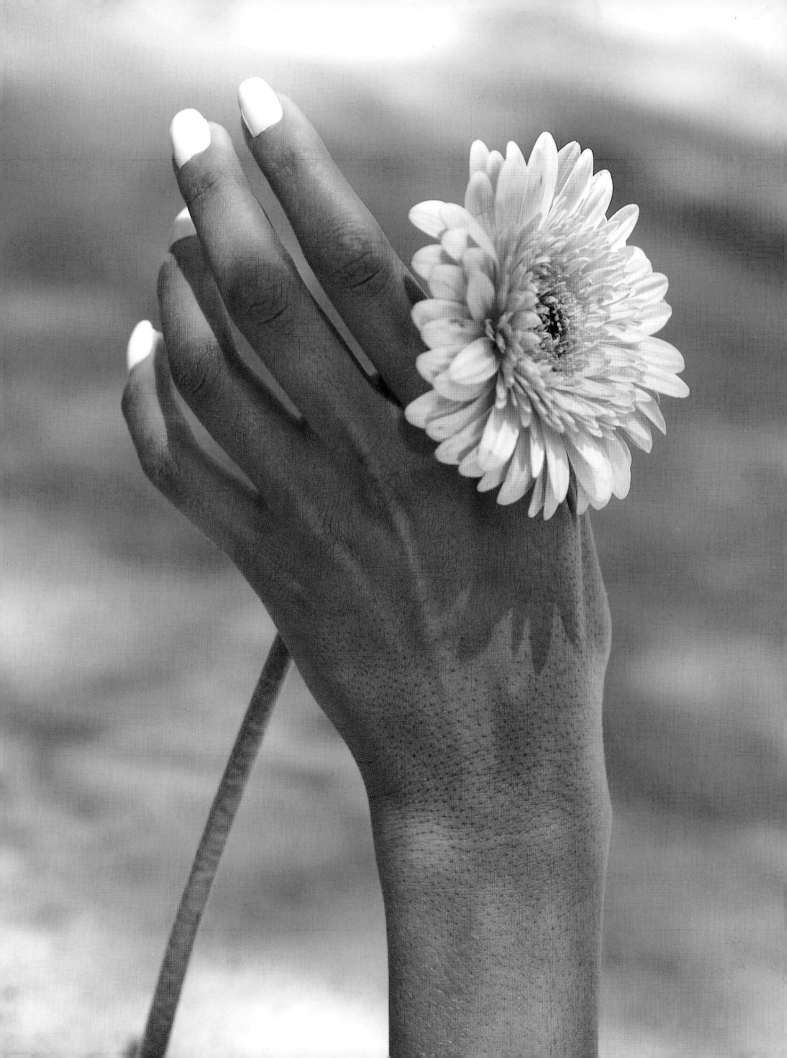

Gel nails

Gel nails are created by applying layers of gel acrylic to the nails. These combine and harden to form a solid nail. Depending on the formula used, nails are hardened with an ultraviolet light or under ordinary room lighting. Gels are among the most natural-looking of all nail enhancements and worth thinking about if you want nails that look like your own, only longer and stronger. Get a nail technician to apply your gel nails for you as doing it yourself is tricky. That said, the basic steps are outlined here to help you understand the process.

Method 1: Fibre wraps

1 Natural nail surfaces are buffed and free edges filed to shape. A drop of nail adhesive is applied to the nail tip, which is held at a 45-degree angle. The top of the tip is placed at the free edge, rolled back, pressed down and held till secure.

2 The tips are trimmed with a special nail tip trimmer.

3 The tips are shaped with a nail file and any rough edges are smoothed away.

4 The tip seam is blended where it joins the nail and the free edge is shaped with a medium to fine file.

5 Nails are buffed and smoothed carefully.

6 The self-adhesive microfibre wrap is applied.

7 One to two coats of thin acrylic gel are applied to the wraps and allowed to set.

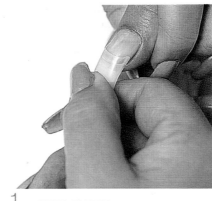

1 ATTACH TIP

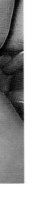

2 TRIM TIP

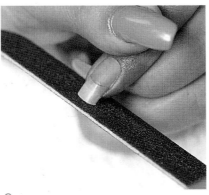

3 FILE TIPS TO SHAPE

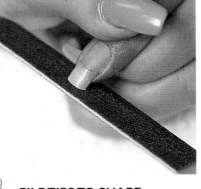

4 BLEND TIPS

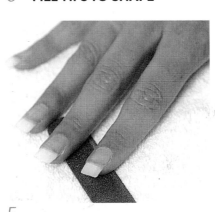

5 BUFF AND SMOOTH

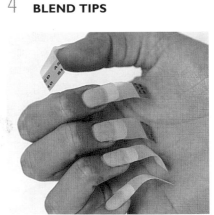

6 APPLY MICROFIBRE WRAP

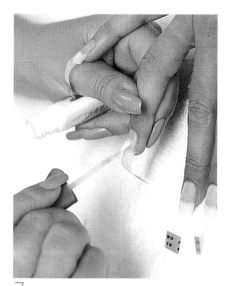

7 **APPLY THIN ACRYLIC**

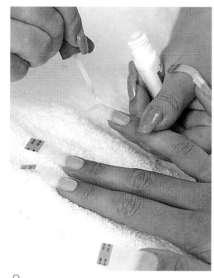

8 **BUILD CONTOURS**

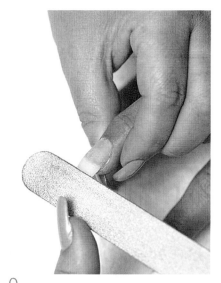

9 **FILE AND BUFF**

8 When dry, the remnants of the fibre wraps are cut away and any roughness filed smooth. Thick acrylic gel is applied to build up the nail contours.

9 Once set, nails are filed and buffed, and topcoat applied.

TIPS

- **Enhancements need 'filling' every two to four weeks, depending on how quickly your nails grow. The area next to the cuticle is filled by the technician to match the rest of the nail.**
- **When any enhancements are removed, your natural nails may be paper thin.**

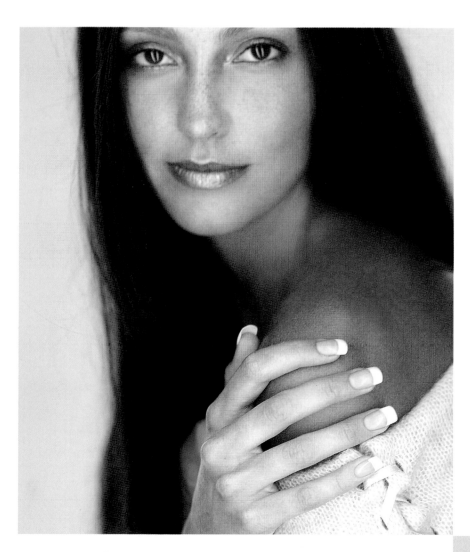

Method 2: **Acrylic overlay**

1 The natural nail surfaces are buffed with a buffer to remove shine only, then the free edge of the nail plate is filed to shape. One drop of nail adhesive is applied to the nail tip, which is held at a 45-degree angle and positioned correctly by placing the top of the tip at the free edge. Then the tip is rolled back and pressed down, holding it in place for a few seconds until it is secure.

2 One coat of acrylic bonding agent is applied to the natural nail only.

3 Acrylic is applied using the ball method: The brush is dipped into the liquid and pressed against the dish to release any excess. The tip of the brush is swept across the surface of the powder until it has gathered as much powder as it can hold, and is large enough to cover the entire nail. The ball of product is then applied to the centre of the nail.

4 Working quickly while still wet, the acrylic is pushed back to fill in the cuticle area, toward the sides and forward to complete the nail overlay.

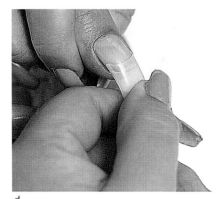

1 **APPLY TIPS**

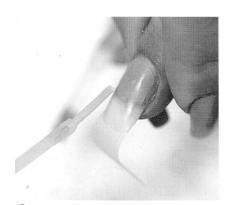

2 **APPLY BONDING AGENT**

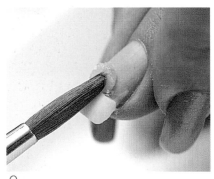

3 **APPLY ACRYLIC**

The nails are tapped, and the nail technician listens for the clicking sound that will indicats that the product has completely cured.

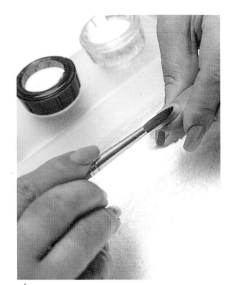

4 **FILL IN**

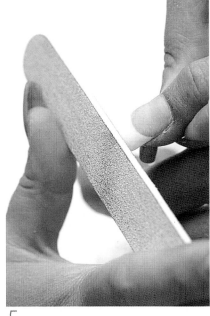

5 **FILE AND BUFF**

5 Nails are filed and buffed, then completed according to your needs – basecoat, polish and topcoat. A drop of cuticle oil is applied to each cuticle.

Method 3: Sculpted acrylic

1 Nails are buffed and sterilized, then sculpted using cutaway disposable paper forms or reusable metal forms.

2 One coat of acrylic bonding agent is applied to the natural nail to help bond the keratin with the polymer.

3 The chosen form is fitted to each finger, ensuring it fits correctly. It is held securely in position during application. If a reusable form (3a) is used, it is slid onto the finger, making sure the free edge of the nail fits over it and it sits snugly. If disposable forms (3b) are used, one is peeled from its paper backing. It is bent into an arch to fit the natural nail shape, slid onto the finger and the adhesive backing is pressed to the sides of the finger. It must fit securely under the free edge and sit level with the natural nail.

4 Acrylic liquid (monomer) and acrylic powder (polymer) are poured into separate glass containers. The brush is dipped into the liquid and pressed against the dish to release any excess.

5 The tip of the brush is swept across the surface of the white acrylic powder until it gathers as much powder as it can hold, and is large enough to shape the entire free-edge extension.

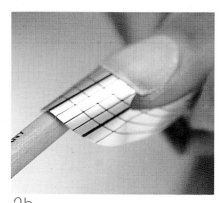

1 **BUFF NAILS**

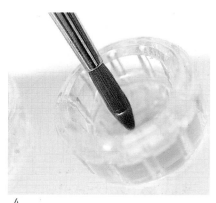

2 **APPLY BONDING AGENT**

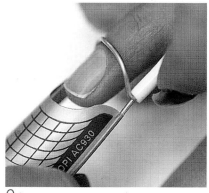

3a **FIT REUSABLE FORM**

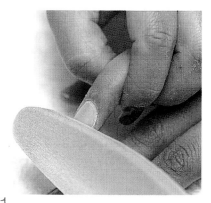

3b **FIT DISPOSABLE FORM**

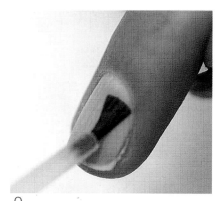

4 **ACRYLIC LIQUID**

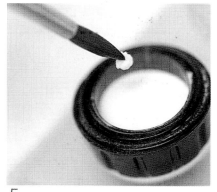

5 **WHITE POWDER**

6 The acrylic ball is placed on the centre of the nail form where it joins the free edge.

7 The acrylic is dabbed, pushed and pressed to shape an extension using the middle portion of the brush.

8 Sides are kept parallel and shaped continuously along the free edge. A dabbing action creates a more natural-looking nail. (If the two-colour acrylic method is used, the natural free-edge line must be followed with the white powder to create a French manicure.)

9 A second ball of acrylic is created using the pink acrylic powder.

10 The second ball of acrylic is placed on the natural nail next to the free edge line in the centre of the nail.

11 The ball is shaped by dabbing and pressing out to the side walls, making sure the product is very thin around all edges.

12 A third ball of pink acrylic is placed at the cuticle area.

13 The ball is smoothed over the nail, gliding the brush over the nail to remove any imperfections. The edges closest to the cuticle, sidewall and free edge must be very thin for the most convincing nails.

14 The nails are tapped with the brush handle to hear if they make a clicking sound. This will indicate that the nails are completely dry.

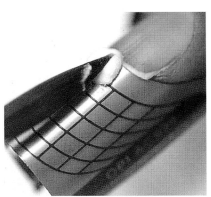

6 **PLACE FIRST BALL**

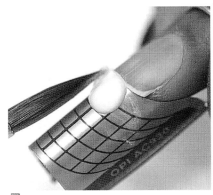

7 **DAB, PUSH AND PRESS**

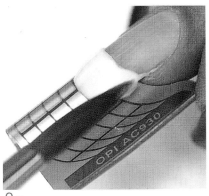

8a **CONTINUE SHAPING**

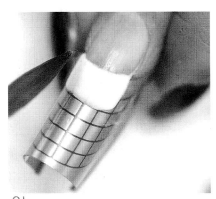

8b **SHAPING COMPLETED**

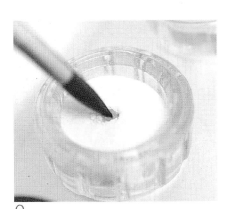

9 **PINK ACRYLIC LIQUID**

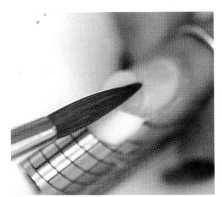

10 **PLACE SECOND BALL**

15 The forms are removed once nails are thoroughly dry.

16 Nails are shaped using a medium-grade emery board, then buffed until the entire surface is smooth.

17 Nails are finished with a layer of basecoat, two coats of nail polish if desired, and a top-coat. Finally, a drop of cuticle oil is applied to each cuticle.

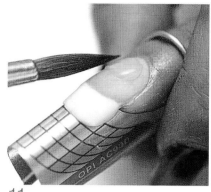

11 **SHAPE ACRYLIC**

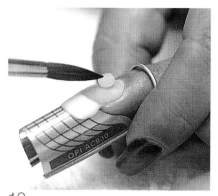

12 **PLACE THIRD BALL**

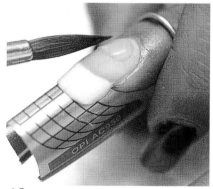

13 **SMOOTH OVER NAIL**

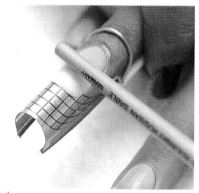

14 **TAP NAIL FOR DRYNESS**

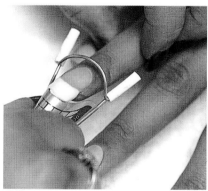

15a **REMOVE METAL FORM**

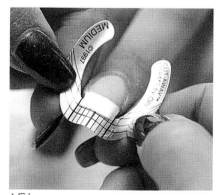

15b **REMOVE DIPOSABLE FORM**

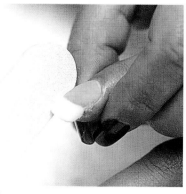

16 **SHAPE NEW NAILS**

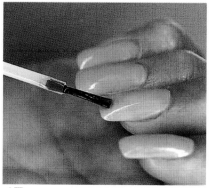

17 **APPLY POLISH**

HANDS 69

Nail tips

Preformed nail tips are attached to the natural nail with nail glue and generally applied halfway down the nail plate. For a smoother finish, some nail technicians may apply acrylics, gels or wraps over either the natural 'untipped' nail or both the natural nail and the new tip. The entire shape is then filed into the length and shape you want. You can buy nail enhancement kits that contain tips but because of the chemicals involved, your best option is to visit a nail technician. The basics are explained here to help you understand the process.

1 The natural nail surfaces are buffed to remove shine and the free edge is filed into shape. One drop of nail adhesive is applied to the nail tip, which is held at a 45-degree angle and positioned correctly by placing the top of the tip at the free edge. The tip is rolled back and pressed down, holding it in place for a few seconds until it is secure.

2 The tip seam is blended and filled with acrylic gel.

3 While still wet, the acrylic is smoothed with a brush.

4 The nails are dried using a specially designed ultraviolet lamp. Later, the nails are buffed and smoothed. They are then finished according to your personal preference – basecoat, two coats of varnish if you choose to use colour, and a topcoat to finish.

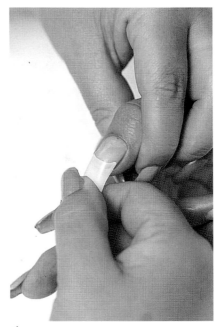

1 **APPLY TIP**

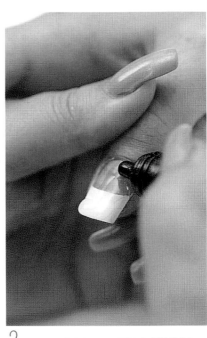

2 **FILL SEAM WITH ACRYLIC**

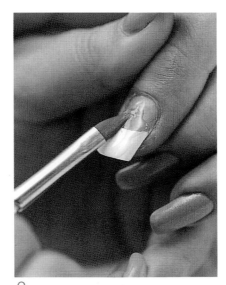

3 **SMOOTH ACRYLIC GEL**

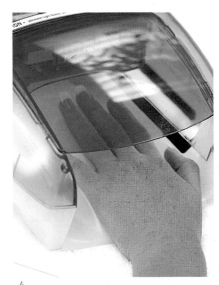

4 **DRY NAILS**

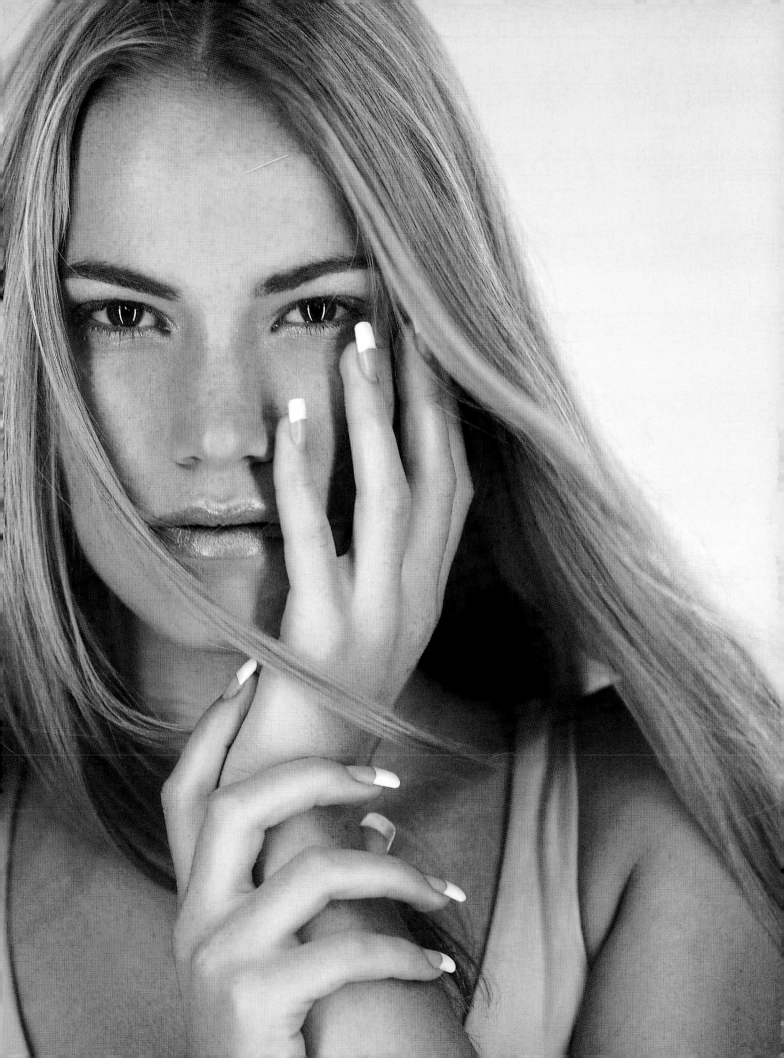

Fashion nails

Get as creative as you like; the choices are endless, with colours in every imaginable spectrum. Do not stick to pinks and reds, but try some of the wilder shades of green, blue, yellow and silver. With all sorts of commercially produced nail adornments from rhinestones and gems, striping tape and transfers, you are spoilt for choice. The photographs on this page show a pretty, commercially produced jewelled nail overlay that is easy to do yourself.

1 Follow the basic manicure steps up to the nail polish application. Apply the basecoat, followed by two coats of your chosen shade of nail polish.

2 Select the correct size decorative nail overlay for each finger, filing your natural nail and the sides of the artificial nail for a perfect fit. Bear in mind that your own nails need to be the same length as the transparent overlay for the desired effect. Carefully apply glue to the overlay.

3 Slowly lower the overlay into place and hold it firmly until it sets. (To remove, file the tips of the overlay to break through the protective top-coat. Then soak your nails in non-acetone-based nail polish remover until soft. Wipe off the softened plastic and glue to reveal your natural nail underneath.)

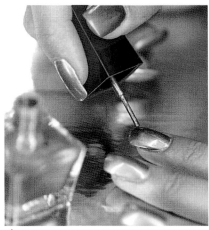

1 **APPLY COLOUR**

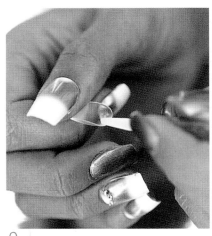

2 **APPLY GLUE**

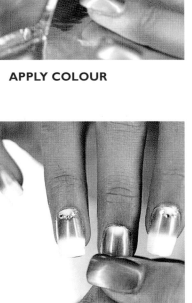

3 **PLACE OVERLAY**

POLISH TIPS

- **Avoid quick-dry polishes, which generally contain acetone that parches your nails. Thicker, slower-drying varnish holds moisture and gives nails more flexibility.**

- **Roll polish bottle in your palms to mix. Never shake – this causes air bubbles and uneven application.**

Below: A. High gloss; B. pearlized; C. glitter appliqué; D. sparkle overlay; E & F. Metallic; G. frosted; H. transparent

A  B   C   D   E   F   G   H

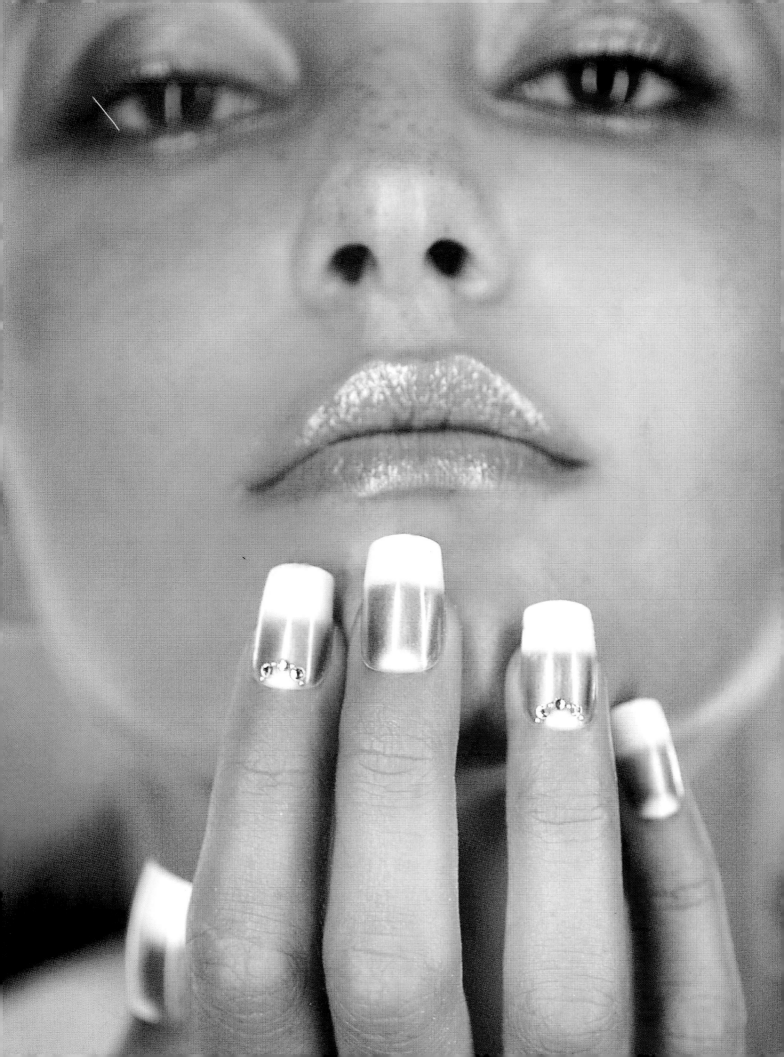

The salon manicure

Nothing beats the indulgence of a salon manicure, especially if you have the time to be pampered. Give yourself a treat – simply relax and put yourself in the hands of a professional.

1 Old nail varnish is removed by swiping it off with a piece of cotton wool saturated with varnish remover. Nails are rinsed again immediately.

2 Nails are filed into shape and any small imperfections are buffed away.

3 A mild exfoliator is applied to dampened hands, which are gently massaged. The exfoliator is rinsed off and the hands are dried thoroughly.

4 Hands are soaked in soapy water for 10 minutes.

5 Cuticles are moisturized with a cuticle cream.

6 Cuticles are gently pushed back using a hoof stick.

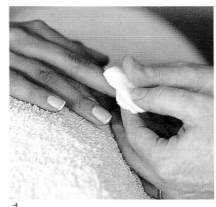
1 REMOVE OLD VARNISH

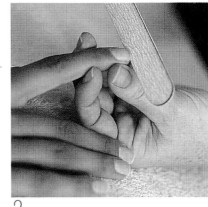
2 FILE NAILS

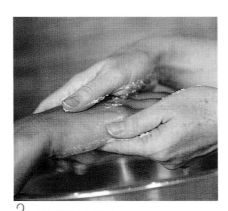
3 EXFOLIATE

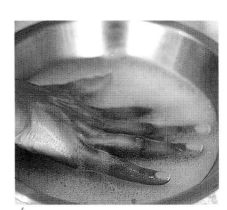
4 SOAK HANDS

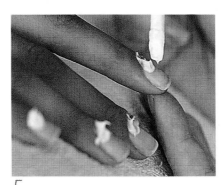
5 MOISTURIZE CUTICLES

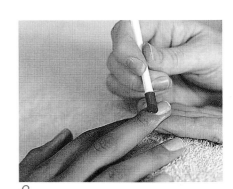
6 PUSH BACK CUTICLES

7 Cuticles and hands are massaged to ensure the hand cream is absorbed.

8 Excess dead skin and hangnails are trimmed with small sharp nippers, ensuring that no living skin is cut.

9 Nails are buffed to remove any unevenness, imperfections or ridges.

10 Arms and hands are massaged with rich moisturizing cream.

11 Hands are submerged in a warm, nourishing vitamin E paraffin bath. Paraffin wax traps in heat and moisture and opens the pores of the skin. Hands are dipped a few times, with a few seconds in-between each immersion, so that the wax builds up in layers. The hands are then wrapped in plastic bags and slipped into insulated terry towelling mitts. After 10 minutes, the wax is peeled off, leaving hands soft.

12 Nail varnish is applied according to your requirements – first the basecoat, followed by two layers of the nail varnish of your choice, and finally the topcoat to seal and protect.

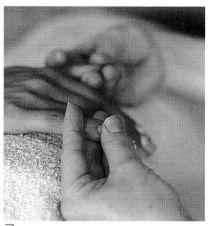

7 **MASSAGE IN CREAM**

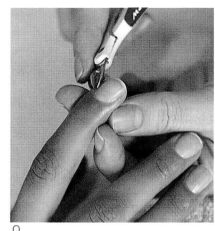

8 **TRIM HANGNAILS**

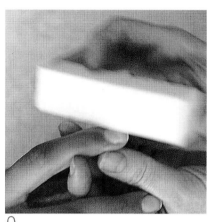

9 **BUFF NAILS**

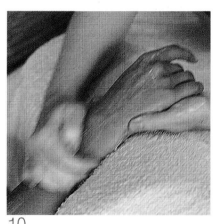

10 **MASSAGE**

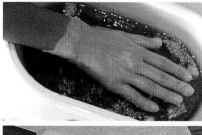

11 **WAX AND WRAP**

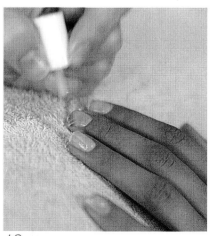

12 **VARNISH**

Spa treat

Escapism is all-important to the spa concept. However, while spas offer a once-in-a-while retreat, not many of us can manage to book into a hydro, so creating a sanctuary within your own space is the key to long-term stress survival. Aromatherapy oils, indulgent scrubs, scented candles and a pile of fluffy towels can do wonders for the soul, not to mention your hands. With a little imagination, a spa moment can happen at any time in any place.

1 Soak hands in a herbal or floral infusion, such as lavender, neroli or geranium, to revitalize and reduce fatigue.

2 Wash and scrub hands using an indulgent soap or suitable handwash. If your hands are grimy and stained, scrub them gently with a bristle nailbrush. Gently dry each nail in turn with a fluffy towel.

3 Gently ease away stress and strain by treating yourself to a gentle reflexology massage (*see* pages 24–25). Or, follow the basic massage guide on pages 78–79.

4 Make your own hand and foot scrub by combining one cup of sea-salt, one cup of massage oil or olive oil, and six drops of stimulating essential oil. Gently rub this over your hands to remove rough skin and boost circulation.

5 Masks are a good way to rev up the skin in no time at all. Cleansing masks, which often contain fruit extracts or clay, absorb excess oils. Some moisturizing masks also contain toning and firming ingredients such as seaweed, herbs and aromatherapy oils. Slather the mask liberally onto the back of your hands and leave it on for as long as indicated in the instructions. Rinse it off and pat the hands dry.

6 Apply hand lotion and massage into hands and arms to finish off your spa treat.

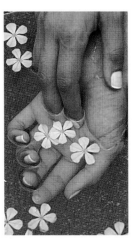
1 **SOAK**

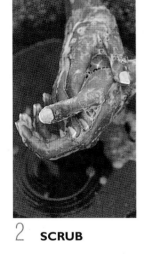
2 **SCRUB**

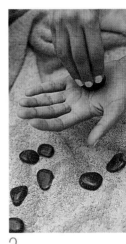
3 **MASSAGE**

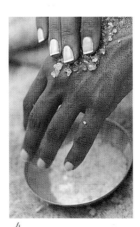
4 **EXFOLIATE**

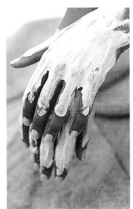
5 **MASK**

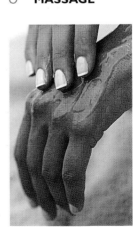
6 **MOISTURIZE**

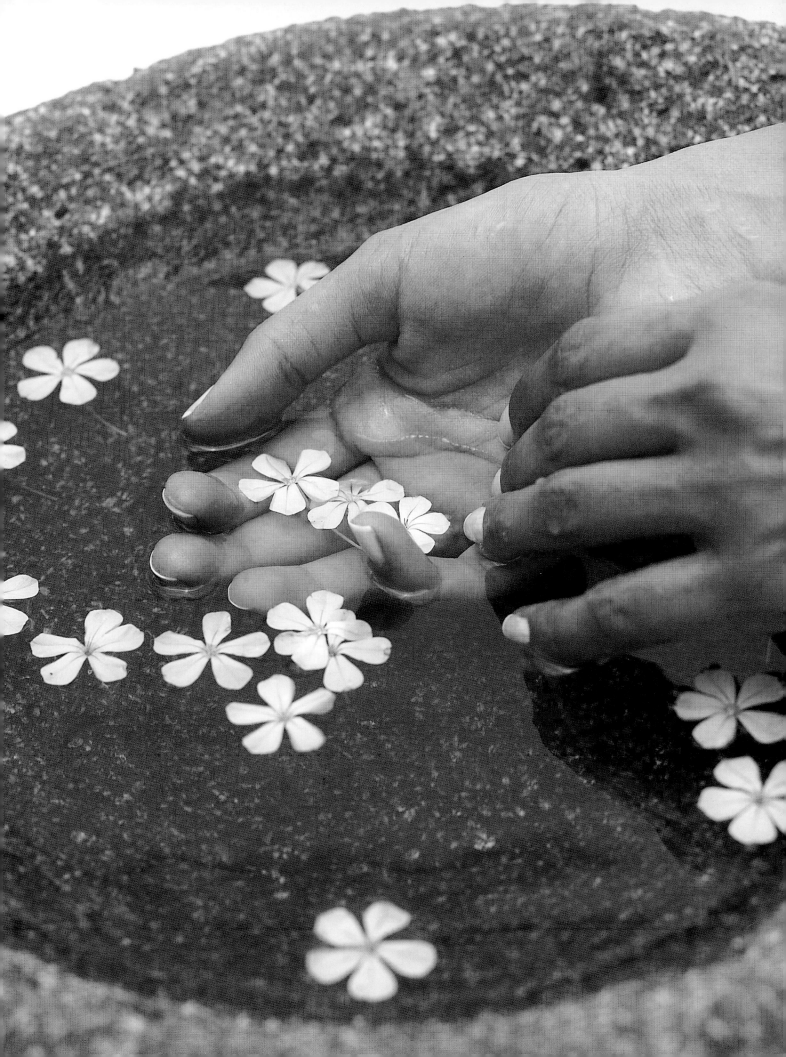

Massage basics

Massage is the ultimate feel-good destressor, great for relaxing tired muscles and improving circulation. Here are some basic DIY massage techniques to tone and stretch your muscles, boost circulation and limber up your joints.

1 Rub on some moisturizing cream or add a few drops of a pure essential oil to a carrier oil, such as almond oil. Rub your palms together briskly to create warmth, then spread the oil over each hand, rubbing the palm of one hand over the back of the other, as if you were washing your hands.

2 Using the thumb and index finger of one hand, work the other palm and upper hand in circular kneading motions. Next, grasp each finger and gently pull from the joint to the fingertips, finishing off by massaging the knuckles. Repeat on the other hand.

3 Place four fingers of your right hand on the back of the left hand, keeping the right thumb free to work on your left palm. Bend the thumb, and in a rotating movement gently press the thumb clockwise or anticlockwise, moving over the entire palm of the left hand as you work. Repeat with the left thumb on the palm of the right hand.

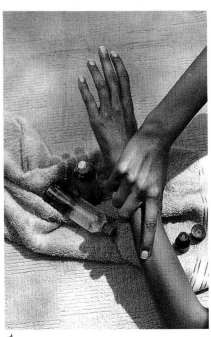

1 **RUB ON CREAM/OIL**

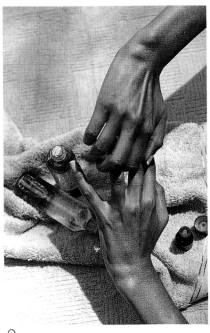

2 **PULL FINGERS**

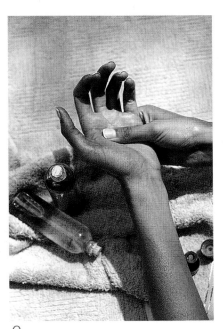

3 **RUB THE PALM**

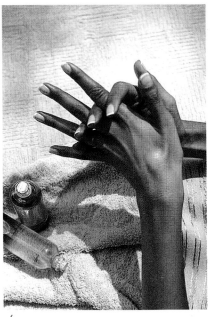

4 **SLIDE FINGERS**

4 With fingers outstretched and intertwined, slide the fingers of one hand firmly up and down the other, with palms facing. Slowly turn the palms outward, stretching your arms in front of you for an easy stretch.

5 With the index and middle fingers of your right hand, gently 'milk' each finger as if you were milking a cow. Begin closer to the knuckle and gently but firmly pull, squeeze and work your way down to the tips of each finger. Repeat, using the fingers of your left hand to massage your right hand.

6 Massage the left elbow and forearm with the fingers of your right hand, using circular movements from the elbow all the way down to the wrist. Knead the outer muscle of the forearm, working slowly up and down the arm. Repeat on the right arm. To complete the massage, release and shake out your hands as if you were drying your nails.

Below: Oils help to provide lubrication for your massage.

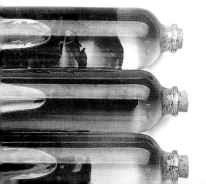

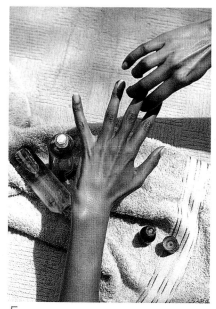

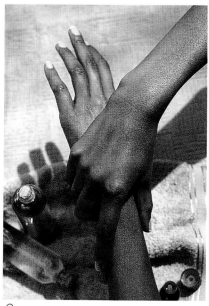

5 **'MILK' FINGERS**

6 **MASSAGE FOREARM**

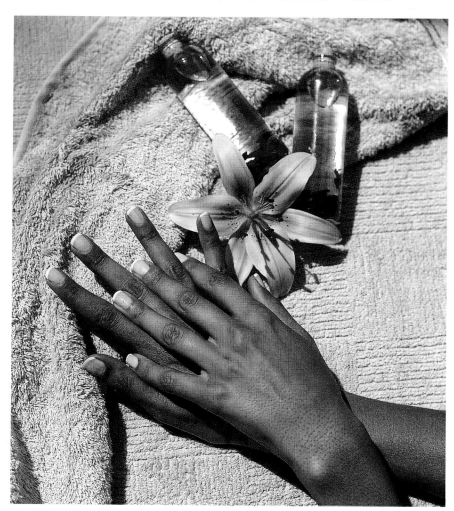

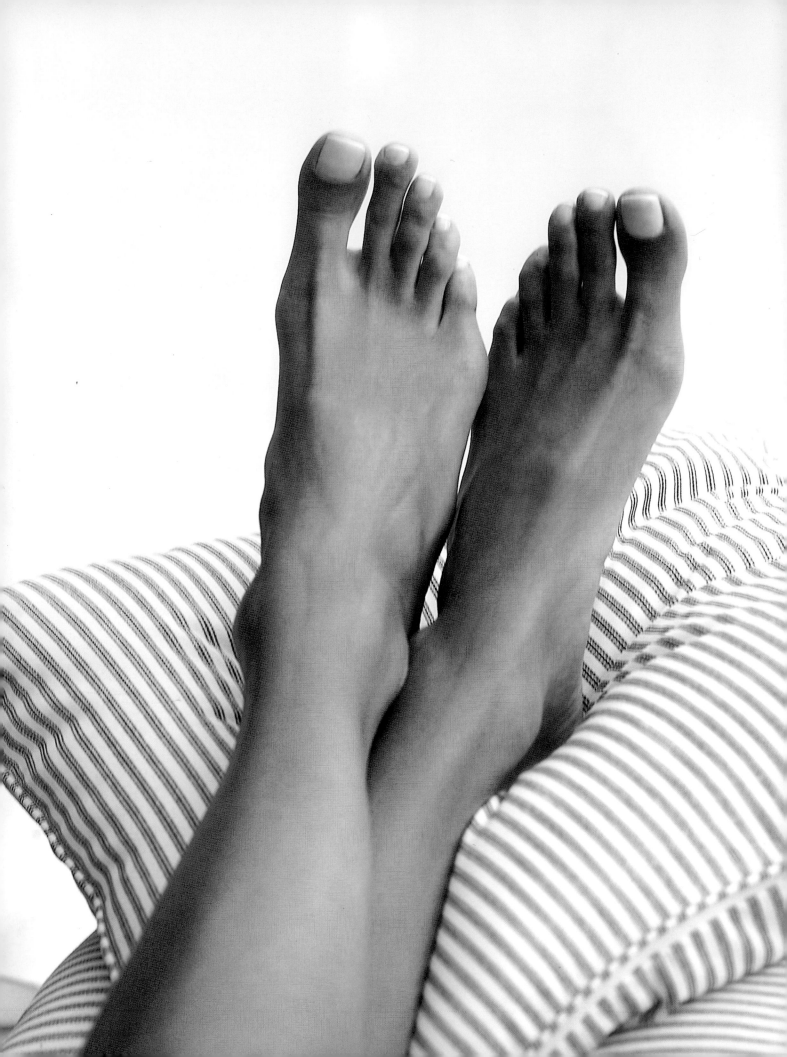

PART TWO

feet

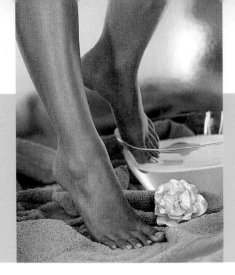

Foot structure and problems

Your feet consist of an amazing framework of bones, ligaments, muscles and tendons designed to bear the weight of your body efficiently and enable mobility. Together, your feet contain 52 bones – a quarter of the bones in your body – as well as 33 joints, 112 ligaments and a complicated network of blood vessels, tendons and nerves. Together, these enable you to move fluidly and with balance.

Amazingly, on the relatively small area of the feet manage to support some 45–112kg (100–250lbs) of body weight.

The feet also act as the body's shock absorbers, and as levers to propel the body forward when you walk or run.

The structure of the foot is similar to that of the hand, but the toes lack the mobility of the thumb and fingers. The heel pad and arches of the foot act as shock absorbers, cushioning the impact of each step. This is necessary because basic wear and tear caused by the simplest chores exerts several thousand tons of pressure onto your feet every day. It is estimated that the average person takes approximately 8000 steps per day. By the time you are 70, you will have covered a distance equivalent to walking around the world three times.

Modern lifestyles place further strain on the feet in the form of hard surfaces, poor exercise, increased work stress and poorly designed fashion footwear. Together with wear and tear that comes with age, injury and disease, these are the hidden causes of many foot problems. Since feet experience more wear and tear than other parts of the body, they are prone to injury. Of all physical ailments, foot problems are probably the most common.

Right: Avoid narrow, pointed shoes, which can damage the structure of your feet.

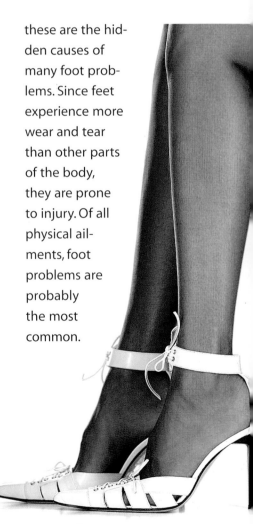

Foot shape, size, arch height and toe lengths are an inherited combination from your parents, which may predispose you to foot problems, such as bunions or high arches.

Muscles of the lower leg and foot

Each foot contains 19 muscles. Although these muscles are small, they must provide support and cushioning for both the foot and the entire leg.

The *extensor digitorum longus* at the side of the calf bends the foot up and extends the toes, whereas the *tibialis anterior* at the front of the shin bends the foot upward and inward.

The *peroneus longus* on the outer side of the calf is the muscle that inverts the foot and turns it outward. The *peroneus brevis*, origi-nating on the lower surface of the fibula (calf bone), serves to bend the foot down and outward.

The *gastrocnemius*, attached to the lower rear surface of the heel, pulls the foot down, while the *soleus*, which originates at the upper portion of the fibula, also helps to bend the foot down.

Muscles in the foot – including the *extensor digitorum brevis, abductor hallucis, flexor digitorum brevis* and the *abductor* – move the toes and help you to main-tain balance while walking and standing.

STRUCTURE OF THE FOOT

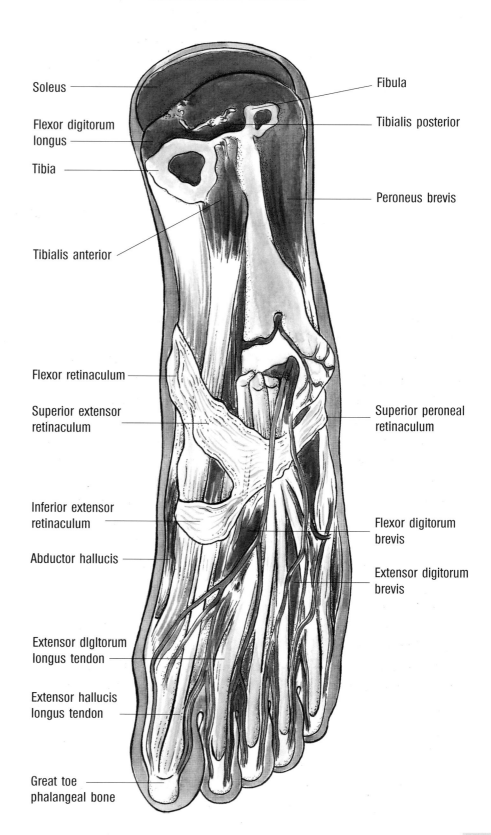

Soleus

Flexor digitorum longus

Tibia

Tibialis anterior

Flexor retinaculum

Superior extensor retinaculum

Inferior extensor retinaculum

Abductor hallucis

Extensor digitorum longus tendon

Extensor hallucis longus tendon

Great toe phalangeal bone

Fibula

Tibialis posterior

Peroneus brevis

Superior peroneal retinaculum

Flexor digitorum brevis

Extensor digitorum brevis

Understanding foot problems

In supporting the weight of the body, the feet have to take considerable strain. To cope with this, they have a complex structure of bones, muscles, sinews and nerves. Each foot contains 26 small, delicate bones – the highest concentration of bones of any structure in the human body. To keep them in their correct position and provide elasticity, there are four times as many ligaments and muscles as there are bones. All of these need to be looked after if they are to work properly.

The ankle bones form a tripod (triangular) shape, which gives you balance and mobility. The main strength of the foot comes from the big toe, and your true centre of balance is the ball of the foot.

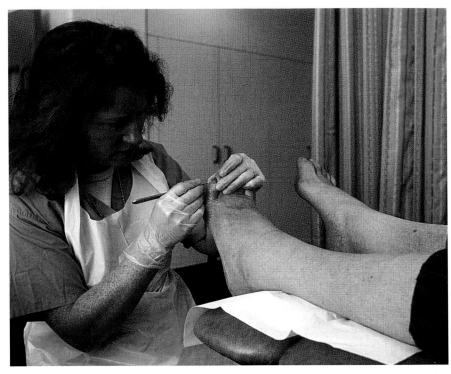

A regular visit to a podiatrist can help to control or prevent foot problems.

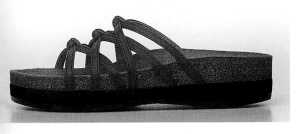

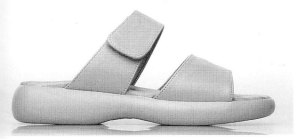

Sensible orthopaedic shoes help to minimize foot disorders.

Apart from bearing the body weight, the feet have a great deal of work to do. In spite of this, they are – together with the hands – among the most neglected parts of the body. Any disturbance or inhibition of the foot's structure may result in general health problems, some of the most common being: fallen arches; high arches; weak ankles; bunions; hammer toes; corns; and pain under the heels, arches or toe joints.

For this reason, feet need to be properly supported, and balanced, and protected by good shoes, which are the key to healthy feet. (*See* pages 94–97 for how to choose shoes.) Basic foot care and an occasional pedicure can also

help. There are also many reasons to visit a nail technician; she can smooth your calluses (not to mention your nerves), cleanse your feet, rev up your circulation and shape your toenails.

If a foot is not functioning correctly, it can affect the alignment and function of the knees, hips, spine and shoulders, causing pain or loss of mobility. The body is very delicately balanced; a slight impairment of proper function in the foot will throw everything else out of balance. Over time, this may result in damage to joints, bones and tendons. Fatigue and irritability – even headaches – can be related to problems with your feet.

Other health conditions requiring foot care include diabetes, arthritis, poor circulation, differences in the length of your legs, work and sporting injuries, and nervous conditions such as spasticity and cerebral palsy.

Poor circulation, for example, requires special foot care as it slows the healing process so small irritations such as cuts, bruises, blisters, corns or calluses, have the potential to become infections, open sores and ulcers. Never try harsh home treatments such as cutting corns and calluses, which could cause bleeding.

Diabetics cannot process carbohydrates effectively, resulting in abnormal blood sugar levels. They often suffer from athlete's foot as their perspiration is sweet from increased blood sugar, providing a breeding ground for fungus. Diabetics should visit a foot specialist at least twice a year in order to prevent minor problems becoming major ones, particularly as they may experience gradual loss of nerve function in the legs and feet. This decreases their capacity to notice if the foot is injured, or if ulcers are forming.

If you ignore foot problems, they may deteriorate and require more invasive treatment.

Remember that prevention is better than cure and that regular visits to a podiatrist or foot specialist will stand you in good stead for years to come.

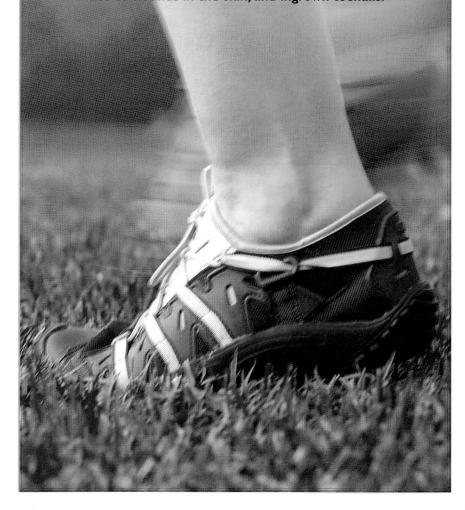

TIPS FOR HEALTHY FEET

- **Wear shoes that fit properly, with enough space not to constrict your toes (see pages 96–97).**
- **Watch the way your shoes are wearing on the soles and heels. If this is uneven, it could indicate a problem with your gait.**
- **Exercise and massage your feet each day.**
- **Take a daily walk in lace-up footwear that is well balanced and supportive. Wear cotton or wool socks rather than manmade fibres; they will keep feet fresh for longer, help prevent blisters, and reduce the risk of fungal growth.**
- **Examine your feet regularly, checking for corns, calluses, athlete's foot, swelling in any of the bones or joints, abnormalities or wounds in the skin, and ingrown toenails.**

Common foot disorders

Athlete's foot

This fungal infection is most commonly seen on the feet of athletes who spend much time in locker rooms, showers and steam rooms. It often starts between the little toes. Symptoms include intense itching, dryness, and mildly red and scaly skin. If the infection is allowed to progress without treatment, blisters may appear.

Treatment requires perseverance; it should be continued over a period of several weeks.

If athlete's foot occurs on a dry area, such as your heel, restore moisture by applying an antifungal cream or ointment. Wash hands thoroughly afterwards to prevent the infection from spreading.

Moist conditions require different treatment: dry feet thoroughly every time you wash; rethink your foot hygiene; wash with cold water instead of hot, which encourages fungal breeding; and apply surgical spirits regularly.

If your treatment regime fails, ask a podiatrist to ensure you are using the best treatment for your particular type of athlete's foot. Several other skin problems can masquerade as athlete's foot; your GP can prescribe a broad-spectrum oral antifungal medication.

Be aware of any symptoms that develop and ensure that you deal with them immediately.

Here are some tips:
• Rotate your shoes to ensure they dry out thoroughly. Frequent sock changes will also help.
• Avoid applying antifungal powder in damp places such as between your toes; it will cake up and irritate your skin. Rather sprinkle the powder inside shoes and trainers. Surgical spirits also help to evaporate the moisture and allow skin to heal.
• Do not rub your feet dry as this removes any new skin; rather pat any moisture away with a towel or disposable paper towel.
• Avoid using moisturizer between your toes; even though the skin is dry and flaky, you need to eliminate any moisture.
• Maintain your shoe rotation, your daily health routine and all treatments even when symptoms vanish. Continue treatment for several weeks after the infection clears as the fungus lies dormant and will reappear if the right conditions present themselves.

Bunions

A bunion, or *Hallux valgus*, is an inflammation and thickening of the joint of the big toe, caused by the big toe being angled excessively toward the second toe. The bunion itself is a symptom of the deformity and can form a large sac of fluid, known as a bursa. Often inflamed and sore, it is aggravated by tight shoes and excessive weight load. If ignored, a bunion will progressively increase in size and become painful.

Women are more prone to bunions than men, partly due to the narrow toe-boxes of fashionable shoes that force the toes into a tapered point. If bunions run in

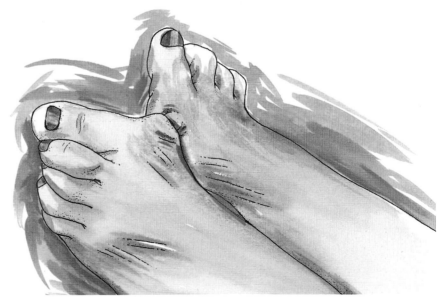

BUNIONS

your family, reduce your risk of following in granny's footsteps by wearing well-fitting, low-heeled shoes with a wide toe-box to accommodate the bunioned foot and remove the source of pressure. If you are not prepared to stop wearing restrictive shoe styles, the bunion will get larger and become painful. Try placing a pad over it to minimize friction.

In addition, talk to your podiatrist, who might recommend exercise, orthoses (special devices inserted into your shoes) or shoe alterations. If necessary, a bunion can be surgically removed.

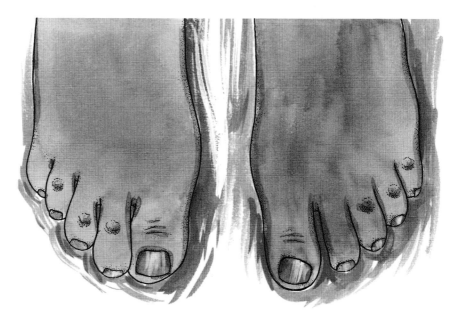

HARD CORNS

Calluses

Calluses are thickened, raised layers of hard, dead skin that form on your feet from repeated friction and pressure where your feet rub against your shoes. When the pressure becomes excessive, some areas of skin thicken and form corns and calluses as a protective response. They can be formed if you wear shoes that are too tight or too short, or even if you walk barefoot a lot.

Calluses can become painful if they are allowed to grow too thick. Use a pumice stone, foot file or chiropody sponge three times a week to rub away hard skin after you have soaked in the bath. Then, follow up with an emollient cream to boost your skin's natural elasticity and delay the callus from building up.

If your calluses are not responding to home treatment, consult a professional. If it feels as though you are 'walking on stones', a podiatrist will remove hard skin, relieve pain and redistribute pressure with a corrective device that fits into your shoes. He or she will also advise you on how to prevent it from happening again.

The best advice on how to avoid these protective calluses from becoming a problem is to take care of your feet: wear shoes that fit; never cut or scrape calluses; and avoid walking on hard concrete surfaces for long periods.

Corns

As already explained, corns and calluses are a build-up of dead skin in a small area as a result of pressure and friction. Unlike calluses, however, corns are usually found over a bony protuberance, such as a joint or bone.

There are five different types, with hard and soft corns being the most common.

• **Hard corns** are the most common, comprising a tough, cone-shaped thickening of the skin, usually within a thickened area of skin or callus. They often have a nucleus in the centre, surrounded by inflamed skin.

• **Soft corns** are usually found between the toes as a result of friction. They are whitish, soggy and rubbery in texture as a result of the sweat or moisture between the toes, which softens the normally hard tissue. Dry your feet thoroughly. A podiatrist might suggest an astringent chemical to help minimize moisture retention.

- **Seed corns** are usually tiny and painless, occur either singly or in clusters underneath the foot, and generally take longer to grow back than other corns. They are formed by callus build-up around cholesterol beads or other anomalies in the sole of the foot.
- **Vascular corns** are either hard or soft corns that also contain blood vessels, which are forced into the growing corn by the squeezing or pinching effect of your shoes. They will bleed profusely if cut and can be exceptionally painful.
- **Neuro-vascular corns** are similar to vascular corns but with both nerve tissue and blood vessels within the growing corn. They often become inflamed and can be very painful.
- **Fibrous corns** result from corns that have been present for a long time. They appear to be more firmly attached to the deeper tissues than other corns, and may be painful.

Self-treatment of corns is not a good idea, especially if you are elderly or diabetic. You could try using a pumice stone to remove the thickened skin a little at a time. Alternatively, use specially designed corn pads to form a protective cushion between the corn and your shoe. However, avoid using corn plasters or paints as these contain caustic chemicals that can damage the healthy tissue around the corns.

Avoid wearing shoes that are too tight, too loose, or have very high heels. Once you relieve the pressure and friction, the corn should gradually start to disappear . Consult your podiatrist, who will be able to remove the corn painlessly and apply padding or prescribe insoles to help minimize pressure, as well as to assist with advice on long-term relief.

Heel pain

The heel bone is the largest bone in the foot. It provides firm support for your body weight and absorbs shock and pressure when your feet hit the ground.

Heel pain can be disabling, making each step a problem, even affecting posture. The most common types of heel pain are:

- **Heel spur:** This develops as an abnormal growth of the heel bone and feels like a painful bruise. Calcium deposits form when the plantar fascia – which is a broad band of fibrous tissue along the bottom of the foot – pulls away from the heel area, causing a bony protrusion, or heel spur, to develop. This injury may cause bone growth to project into the flesh of the foot.

Heel spurs can cause extreme pain, especially when you are standing or walking.

Your podiatrist may apply padding to alter the ligaments' direction of stretch, or apply deep-heat therapy to encourage healing. Alternatively, he or she may decide to prescribe special insoles (orthoses) to help your feet function more effectively and prevent recurrence.

- **Heel bursitis:** This is a constant irritation, resulting in inflammation of the heel's natural cushion (bursa). It is caused by chronic overuse, trauma, rheumatoid arthritis, gout or infection. Pain is felt at the back of the heel when you move the ankle joint, or deep inside the heel when it touches the ground.

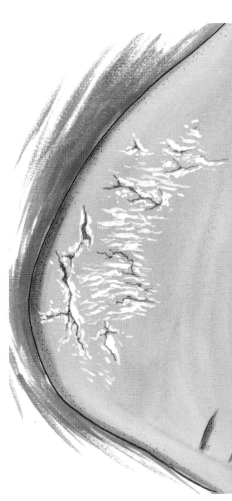

DRY CRACKED HEELS

Immobilization of the affected area, anti-inflammatory medication, the correct orthoses, and cold compresses can be useful to reduce swelling. If not, pay attention to the cause of any rubbing, and get your podiatrist to pad and strap it appropriately. If it is infected, your doctor may need to prescribe antibiotics or to aspirate fluid from the bursa.

• **Heel bumps:** These are recognizable as firm bumps at the back of your heel where the Achilles tendon attaches to the bone. They are aggravated by shoe friction. Mules and slingbacks will help to avoid exerting any pressure on the heel. If pain persists, surgery may be necessary.

Dry, cracked heels

Dry skin often leads to painful cracking of the skin, particularly around the edges of the heels. For many, this may simply be unsightly, but when the fissures are deep, the skin bleeds easily and is painful.

Open-backed shoes, where the rim of the sole causes irritation, may aggravate the condition. Using very hot water can also be a contributing factor.

Use an emollient moisturizing cream on the affected heels daily (look for urea on the list of ingredients). Gentle use of a pumice stone or foot rasp will also help, but never try to pare down the hard skin yourself with a razor blade or a pair of scissors!

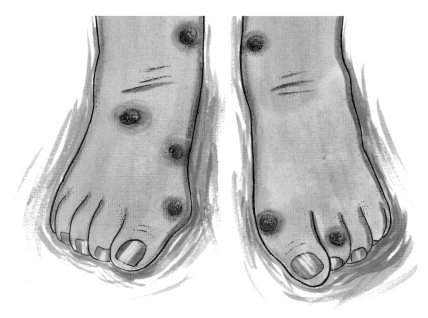

CHILBLAINS

Chilblains

Chilblains are small itchy, red swellings on the skin, which become painful when exposed to damp and cold. As they swell and the surface of the skin cracks open, sores (ulcers) may develop and may become infected.

Chilblains are the result of your skin's abnormal reaction to cold. They occur on the toes, particularly the smaller ones, and sometimes on the face and fingers. They can also occur on areas of the feet that are exposed to pressure – for instance, on a bunion or where your toes are squeezed by tight-fitting shoes.

Many people suffer from cold feet in winter, but whether or not they develop chilblains depends largely on the efficiency of their blood circulation. Draughty or damp conditions, as well as dietary factors and hormonal imbalances can also play a role. To prevent chilblains , a course of calcium before winter may be helpful.

Keep your body, feet and legs warm, especially if your circulation is poor and your mobility is limited. The whole body should be kept warm, not just the feet; trousers, long boots, tights and leg warmers or long socks will help. However, avoid warming chilled skin too rapidly next to a fire or hot-water bottle as this can in fact exacerbate the problem.

Do not scratch chilblains; soothing lotions such as witch-hazel or calamine will take away most of the discomfort. If the chilblain has ulcerated, apply an antiseptic dressing. If you have diabetes or are undergoing medical treatment, have the ulcer assessed by your GP or podiatrist.

Sweaty feet

There are some 250,000 sweat glands in our feet, more per centimetre than anywhere else in the body. They release nearly a cup of moisture every day.

Most people suffer periodically from excessive perspiration and foot odour, yet for some sweaty feet are an embarrassing, persistent problem. Hyperhydrosis (excessive sweating) has much to do with how the sweat glands in the feet work. Excessive odour or sweating of the feet is systemic in some cases, such as anaemia or hyperthyroidism (overactive thyroid).

The sweat glands' function is to keep the skin moist and supple. Throughout the average day, the body naturally perspires to regulate heat in the body. Sweaty feet can also be caused by stress on the foot due to a structural problem, or because the foot is under strain or is tired – for example, when you have been standing all day.

Hot weather may aggravate the condition, even though sweaty feet are not only a summer problem. Since sweat glands on the

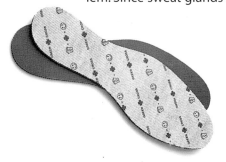

Medicated insoles may help to prevent foot odour.

feet and hands can also be triggered by emotional responses, mental or emotional stress may be a contributing factor. In teenagers, sweaty feet are often triggered by hormonal changes.

Frequently accompanying sweaty feet is foot odour, which occurs when bacteria on the skin break the sweat down. Simple hygiene is usually effective in dealing with this problem:

• Wash your feet daily with anti-bacterial soap to minimize the risk of minor skin infections, athlete's foot or blisters.

• Wear well-fitting shoes made of leather, which allow your feet to 'breathe'. Synthetic fibres contribute to the production of excessive perspiration and promote bacterial growth.

• Always wear socks that absorb moisture well; choose natural fibres like wool, cotton, or wool/cotton blends.

• Do not wear the same pair of shoes every day as sweat is absorbed by insoles and uppers; allow shoes to dry out before wearing them again.

• Detachable insoles that can be washed are a good idea, as are medicated insoles, which have a deodorizing effect.

Blisters

A friction blister is a raised area of skin filled with fluid, usually formed between the outer and inner layers of the skin. Blisters

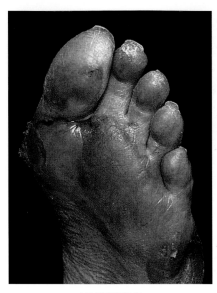

BLISTERS

form as a result of heat, moisture, friction and pressure. The friction from walking causes the skin to be dragged back and forth across the underlying tissue. This leads to a tear in the upper layers of the skin, which fills with fluid – a result of leakage from blood vessels under the skin.

Although most commonly caused by wearing ill-fitting shoes or by using inappropriate footwear for a particular activity, blisters can also appear as a result of infections, burns, skin diseases and insect bites.

Blisters start to form when a sock or shoe clings to damp skin. Reduce friction and moisture and you can help to prevent blisters from developing.

Blisters should be left unbroken wherever possible because they provide valuable protection to the

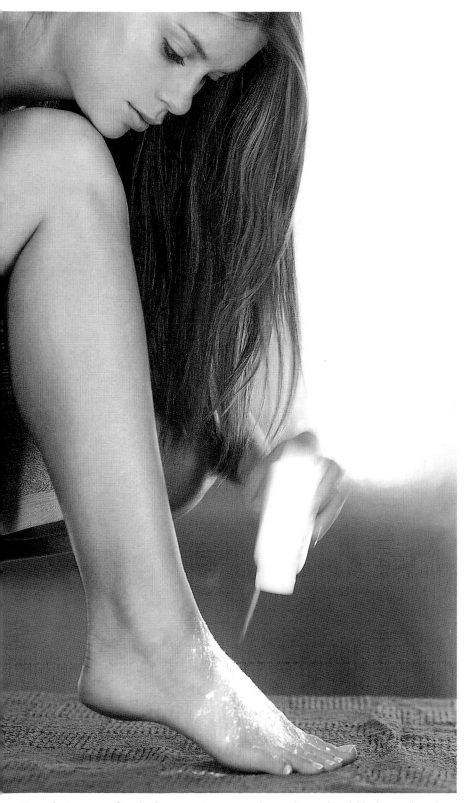

damaged tissue. When a blister has been opened accidentally, always disinfect it with antiseptic and protect it with sterile bandages. Note that blood blisters can result from sharp pinching of the skin when blood collects inside the blister space.

To avoid blisters:

• Buy shoes that fit correctly. Do not forget to allow room for the swelling that is bound to occur as your feet become hot. Add insoles or heel cushions if necessary.

• Wear in new shoes before using them to compete in any sporting activity.

• Consider the type of sock you will wear with the shoe; do not forget that thick socks reduce the volume of a shoe.

• Wear wool or cotton socks that do not bunch up or crease. Wearing two pairs of socks also helps to reduce friction.

• Powder your feet to absorb or reduce moisture and decrease blister-forming friction.

• If the blister continues to cause discomfort, it may need to be lanced and drained. Do not remove the layer of skin covering the blister as this protects the underlying skin from further abrasion. Dress the area with antiseptic ointment, then cover it with a protective plaster.

• Never attempt self-treatment if you have circulatory problems or you are diabetic.

Powdering your feet before putting on socks or shoes should help to absorb any excess moisture that may promote the formation of blisters.

Toenail problems

Your toenails grow 1.6mm to 3mm per month and protect the ends of your toes and the bones and nerves lying underneath. Toenail problems tend to be more common as you get older.

Toenails can suffer a variety of disorders as a result of trauma, disease, ill-fitting shoes, poor hygiene, infection and poor circulation. These problems include bruises, ingrown nails, fungus discoloration, brittleness and curved growth.

Professional care from your podiatrist can help improve the health of your toenails.

Fungal infections

Fingernails and toenails are particularly vulnerable to fungal infections. These occur when fungi (microscopic plants) take up residence in the keratin of your nails. Fungus breeds in dark, damp, warm environments, so avoid walking barefoot in changing rooms or through mud. This affinity for damp, dark places – such as in shoes and socks – is why toenails are more prone to fungal infections than fingernails.

Nails that are brittle, discoloured, dull, abnormally thick, distorted, crumbling, loose, or subject to unusual debris under the nail are a medical rather than a cosmetic problem. They demand the expertise of a dermatologist, podiatrist or medical practitioner.

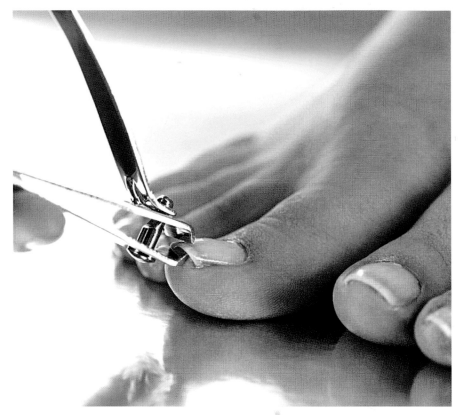

Cut or clip toenails straight across to prevent painful ingrown nails.

Fungal infections are extremely contagious and can be spread through direct contact with contaminated towels, shower and pool surfaces, and nail implements like clippers, orange sticks and cuticle pushers.

People most likely to develop toenail infections include those who frequent public swimming pools, gyms or shower rooms; those who perspire a lot; and those who wear tight shoes.

Symptoms of a nail with fungal infection include discoloration and thickening of the nail, and the separation of the nail from the nail bed. There may be a white, cheesy discharge. Without treatment, the nail bed itself can become infected. Treatment options include antifungal or antibacterial cream, and professional trimming, shaping and care of the nail by your podiatrist. An infection can take as long as seven months to cure, as it must grow out with the nail.

Nail infections do not always respond to topical treatments; if severe, you may need to use oral antibacterial medication.

Ingrown toenails

The most common problem treated by podiatrists is ingrown toenails (or onychocryptosis). The big toe is particularly prone to this painful condition, which occurs when one or two corners of a nail grow into and become embedded in the surrounding skin. It feels like a splinter and can be very painful. In severe cases, it may even cause pus and bleeding.

Most ingrown toenails are self-inflicted as a result of incorrect trimming technique, trauma (such as stubbing your toe), or from wearing tight-fitting shoes, socks or tights that push your toe against the nail so that it pierces the skin.

Try these tips to prevent this painful affliction from recurring:

- Cut toenails straight across so they are even with the tip of the toe. Do not cut too short, too low at the edge or down the side. File any pointed edges smooth with an emery board.
- Avoid using nail cutters as the curved cutting edge may cut the flesh. Nail scissors can also slip so it is best to use nail nippers. These have a smaller cutting blade but a longer handle for ease of use.
- Cut nails after a bath/shower when softer and easier to cut.
- Keep toenails square in shape. Rounding the corners may be prettier, but this only encourages nails to grow into the surrounding skin. File sharp edges slightly to smooth any roughness.

- Avoid toe-pinching shoes. Cramming toes into tight shoes often leads to nail problems. Do not be vain; wear a larger shoe size.
- Practise good hygiene. Rotate your footwear so that each pair of shoes has a chance to dry out thoroughly before you wear them again. Opt for breathable materials and wear natural-fibre socks. In summer, wear open-toed sandals when ever possible.

The treatment of ingrown toenails depends on the severity of the condition.

- If you have a mildly ingrown nail, try to remedy it yourself. Fill a basin with warm water, add a tablespoon of salt and soak your feet for 15 to 20 minutes. Dry thoroughly. Next, gently wedge a tiny bit of cotton wool under the corner of the nail. Repeat this nightly for two or three weeks until the nail has grown out.
- If strong pain, swelling, redness, pus or infection develops around an ingrown toenail, visit your doctor or podiatrist immediately. Remember, never start digging yourself. Apply a sterile dressing if you have a discharge.
- For the most painful and irritable ingrown toenail, your podiatrist will remove the offending spike of nail and cover it with an antiseptic

dressing. If it is too painful to touch, he or she may inject a local anaesthetic before removing the offending portion of the nail. If you have bleeding or discharge from an infection, or even excessive healing flesh around the nail, you will also need antibiotics if you are to get the better of the infection.

- See a foot specialist immediately if you are diabetic.
- If an ingrown toenail is a recurrent problem your doctor may perform a *matrixectomy* (removal of the matrix, the source of the nail growth, along with the edge of the nail). This will result in permanent narrowing of the toenail.

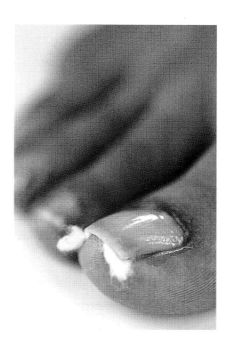

Push cotton wool under an ingrown nail each night to alleviate pressure and encourage correct growth.

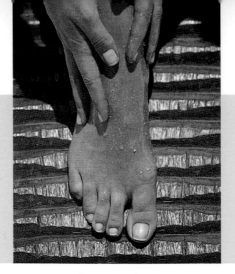

Caring for your feet

For centuries, women have insisted on wearing constricting shoes that contort feet into unnatural positions, so it is not surprising that they are more likely to suffer from foot problems than men. In addition, an average day's walking exerts the equivalent of several hundred tons of pressure on our feet.

Our feet may also suffer from lack of daily hygiene. How many people actually wash and scrub their feet daily, much less dry between the toes? This neglect can lead to foot problems.

Avoiding problems starts with basic foot care, wearing appropriate footwear and giving your feet the occasional pampering treatment. Proper foot care should be as much a part of your daily routine as brushing your teeth. It is never too early – or too late – to start caring for your feet.

Shoe sense

Feet come in all shapes and sizes, even with a choice of types and styles, but how many of us wear shoes best suited to our feet? The 26 bones in each foot are only fully set after we reach 18 years of age, so the shoes we wear as children are crucial to our future foot health. Since some 80 per cent of all foot problems are the result of ill-fitting shoes, it is best to ensure the appropriate fit to guarantee comfortable and healthy feet.

The ideal shoe is 1.5cm (½in) longer than your foot. This is measured from your longest toe, which is often the second toe. The width of the shoe should correspond with the widest part of the foot. It should fit snugly around the heel, over the instep and the big toe. Measure your foot while standing, not sitting, to accommodate the slight spread of the foot when you put your body weight on it. Also remember that your foot swells through the day and needs space to be comfortable.

Ensure your shoes are made of a breathable material, such as leather or fabric, which allow for sweat absorption; avoid synthetic shoes without ample ventilation. Sandals allow air to circulate and do not constrict the toes. A low, broad heel reduces heel pressure.

Choosing shoes that fit properly
Badly fitting shoes can be detrimental to your feet and may even result in backache, sore muscles, fatigue and poor posture. Follow the guidelines on pages 96–97 when buying shoes, and try them on later in the day to allow for the swelling that happens during the day. The perfect shoe should feel comfortable from the moment you try it on.

TOP FOOT-CARE TIPS

1   Wash your feet every day in warm soapy water (do not soak them, which might destroy the natural oils). Dry thoroughly, especially between the toes.

2   If your skin is dry, apply moisturizing cream all over the foot, except between the toes. Moisturizer also helps to avoid painful, cracked heels.

3   Lightly apply foot powder to keep feet dry.

4   Exfoliate your feet regularly. After relaxing in a bath for 10 minutes, gently remove hard skin with a pumice stone, working in small circular motions – except over bony areas or joints, in which case you should consult a podiatrist.

5   Trim your toenails regularly, using nail nippers. Soften nails first by soaking them in warm water or using a softening cream. Cut straight across, not too short, and not down at the corners, which can lead to ingrown nails (see pages 92–93).

6   For a skin-softening treat, smooth a thin film of petroleum jelly onto your feet and wear a pair of cotton socks to bed. The heat generated overnight will intensify the softening properties of the jelly.

7   Give yourself a regular home pedicure (see pages 108–110).

8   Keep feet warm, and exercise them to improve circulation (see pages 99–100).

9   Always wear the right shoe for the job (see the guide to buying shoes on pages 96–97); ill-fitting shoes cause problems.

10   Remember that toenails are more susceptible than fingernails to nail fungus since they tend to be in contact with the ground or are encased in shoes that provide a dark, moist place for bacteria to thrive. Clean, dry feet resist disease; the best way to prevent infection is a strict regimen of washing the feet with soap and water, remembering to dry thoroughly. Wear shower shoes in public areas when possible. Change shoes and socks or hosiery daily.

11   There is no sense in making your toes look pretty if people run away when you remove your shoes! Fight foot odour by cleaning your feet thoroughly every day; changing socks often, sticking with natural fibres such as cotton; using a roll-on antiperspirant to control sweat; wiping your soles with surgical spirit twice a day; and using inserts that contain activated charcoal.

12   Seek prompt treatment for burns, cuts and breaks in the skin, and for any unusual changes in colour or temperature – particularly if you suffer from diabetes.

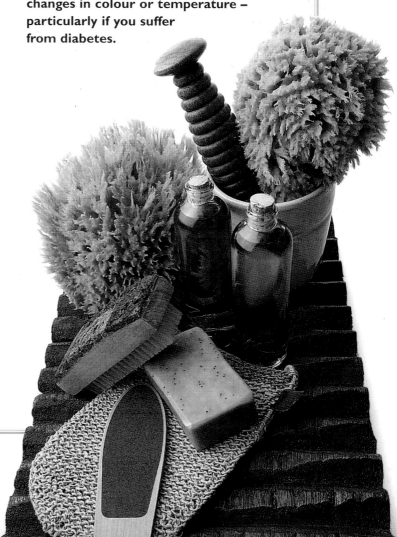

Heel: This carries a large percentage of your weight. The most comfortable heels have a broad base and are no more than 4cm (1½in) in height. Regrettably, heel height is dictated more often than not by the latest fashion rather than comfort levels.

Heel counter: This portion of the shoe cups the heel of the foot around the sides and the back, preventing it from slipping up and down while you walk. Its main function is to stabilize the heel when your foot makes contact with the ground. It should compliment your heel shape. As shoes age and wear, they should be replaced as they generally lose their supporting function. This can lead to foot, leg, and back fatigue, as well as foot problems.

Sole: The underneath of the shoe should be flat, with a slight upward slope under the toes.

Lining: The inner lining should be smooth and free from friction-forming seams that might lead to the formation of blisters.

Upper: This is the main part of the shoe that covers the top of your foot. Ideally, it should be made of a breathable material such as leather, as synthetics without ample ventilation will trap moisture and become smelly.

Fastenings: Ideally, shoes need laces, buckles or Velcro to keep them on your feet. Slip-on shoes offer little support, but renowned health-shoe brands such as

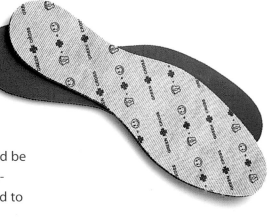

Sole inserts help to cushion the feet.

Birkenstock and Green Cross, although not everyone's aesthetic ideal, allow your feet to breathe, give toes a good gripping workout, and do not constrict the feet in any way.

Choosing sports shoes

Good sports shoes are intended to help your feet perform at peak efficiency while absorbing the shock that is transmitted through the bones, ligaments and tendons with every step. Sportsmen regularly suffer sprains, aches and pains, even fractures, as a result of the overload on their feet that results from inefficient shock-absorption, or even the mechanical inefficiency of the foot.

If you need arch support, motion-control, stability, or cushioning, modern sports shoes help to provide a solution. They are made of high-tech materials that represent millions of dollars worth of research to ensure maximum performance with minimum risk of injury.

PARTS OF A SHOE

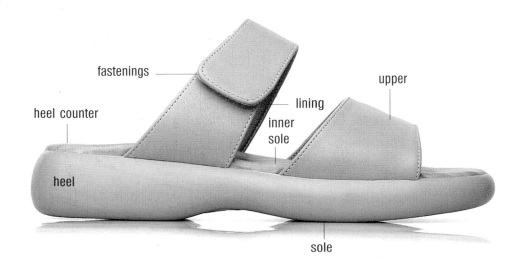

fastenings

heel counter

heel

lining

inner sole

upper

sole

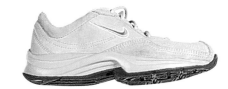

Ladies' walking shoe

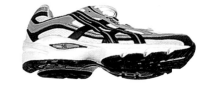

Ladies' running shoe

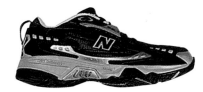

Ladies' cross trainer

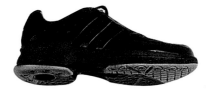

Aerobics shoe

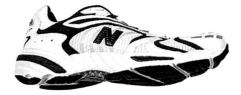

Men's running shoe

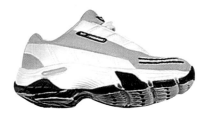

Men's cross trainer

SPORTS SHOES

Running shoes are specifically designed to protect your feet from shock, are very flexible and allow your foot to bend and flex through every step. When you run, the equivalent of three times your body weight is transferred through each foot. As none of this force is absorbed by the ground, the shoe must provide enough shock absorption to prevent damage to feet, legs, ligaments and muscles.

Running involves forward motion rather than stepping sideways – as in tennis, basketball or aerobics – so running shoes are not suitable for activities involving side-to-side movements; their flexibility may give inadequate ankle support when sharp turns or sideways movements are made at speed, resulting in the foot 'going over' at the ankle.

Cross trainers are stiffer in design and ensure greater foot support during side-to-side movements, allowing them to be used for a wider range of activities. There is some loss of flexibility across the ball of the foot and the toes, so muscles and other soft-tissue structures must work harder to bend the foot as you run.

Court shoes, designed for court sports like basketball and tennis, have rubber soles to prevent slipping. They combine flexibility and sideways support.

Fitness shoes, designed for aerobics and similar activities, combine flexibility with support and incorporate cushioning to absorb shock generated during high-impact exercise.

For vanity's sake, most of us wear shoes that are too small for our feet, resulting in ingrown toenails, blisters, even loss of toenails. Sports shoes should feel snug and fit closely around the instep to ensure minimal movement at the heel. The tried-and-tested method of fitting shoes is to check there is space at the end of the shoe by pressing your thumb down in front of the big toe while standing.

If the shoe fits, but you still experience foot problems, consult a podiatrist who deals with foot-related sports injuries or gait problems. He or she might recommend a custom-made insole that fits into the shoe to correct bone and soft tissue misalignment. This will help to treat minor foot problems and prevent them from developing further.

HOT TIPS FROM THE PROFESSIONALS

Nail technician:

- Eliminate dry, rough cuticles by using an exfoliating cuticle treatment containing alpha hydroxy acids twice a week.

- Nail polish removers are very drying; prolong your manicure by applying a new coat of polish over the old at least once before starting afresh.

- Most feet spend 16 hours a day encased in shoes at temperatures as high as 40°C (104°F), resulting in cramped, swollen and fatigued feet. Walk barefoot to exercise feet.

- Regular foot massage helps minimize stress, re-energize, release congestion and toxins and improve circulation.

Podiatrist:

- Remove excess skin daily with a pumice stone or emery board. Cut toenails straight across and never pick or pull toenails.

- Apply an emollient that contains urea (for better absorption) every evening to areas that are dry.

- Choose the correct shoes for your foot structure. Avoid high-heeled, narrow tapering shoes, which can cause havoc with your feet.

- Dry well between the toes and apply talcum powder to help absorb excess moisture.

Therapeutic reflexologist:

- Good comfortable shoes enable your body to cope with the stresses of life and health more effectively. Ill-fitting shoes can aggravate structural problems and bring potential health problems to the fore.

- Walk barefoot regularly to give your body a good workout by stimulating the reflexes and to keep feet supple and mobile.

- Check your feet regularly. Calluses, corns, hard skin and other problems are an indication that your body needs attention.

- Examine your feet for any moles and make sure you consult a dermatologist if you notice that these have changed in any way.

Shoe designer:

- Be meticulous about wearing the correct shoe size: ensure the toe-to-heel length is comfortable, the fitting over the top of the foot is not too tight, and the heel height is comfortable when you are walking.

- Cheap shoes usually compromise on comfort and quality. Avoid plastic shoes/sandals – for the sake of both the condition and odour of your feet.

- The most abusive shoes are strappy high-heeled sandals, which do not offer the required support for your feet. For healthy feet, avoid this type of shoe.

- The least abusive shoe type is the health sandal, which has real leather uppers and a foot bed that supports all the contours of the sole of your foot.

Foot exercises

Just like stomach crunches, foot exercises can shore up weak muscles that may lead to injury. Try these exercises, developed by an orthopaedic surgeon, to help prevent toe cramps, bunions, and hammertoes. Do them barefoot.

1 **Toe stretches:** Sit on a chair, with bare feet on the floor. Raise your heels, keeping toes flat on the floor. Hold for five seconds. Next, roll up onto tips of toes, and hold. Finally, curl tips under, and hold. Return to starting position. Repeat 10 times. This is recommended for people prone to toe cramps or hammer toes, and as a warm-up for strength-training exercises.

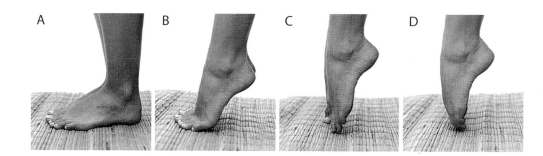

2 **Big-toe pulls:** Place a thick rubber band around both big toes, and pull them away from each other, holding for five seconds. Repeat 10 times. This exercise is good for those with bunions, relieves toe cramp, and helps build muscle.

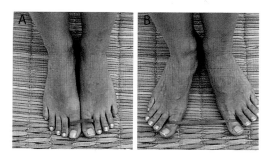

3 **Towel curls:** Place a small towel on the floor near your feet, and pull it up toward you by curling your toes. Repeat five times. Increase the resistance by putting a book or a weight on one end of the towel. This is good for toe cramps and pain in the ball of the foot, on the large outer muscles and the arch.

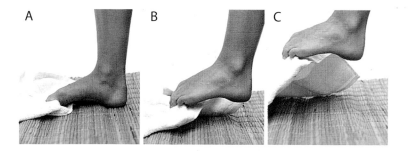

4 **Marble pick-up:** Place 16 to 20 marbles on the floor. Pick up one at a time with your toes, alternating feet. Continue until all marbles are picked up. This exercise tones ligaments and tendons, and isolates and fine-tunes smaller muscles – much as lifting free weights in the gym does.

A   B   C

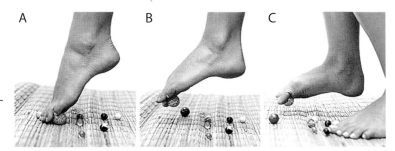

5 **Muscle toner:** Standing on a book or a step, let the toes of both feet hang over the edge, then bend them firmly downward. Hold for a few seconds, then pull them strongly upward, and hold for a few seconds. Repeat the exercise 10 times.

A   B   C

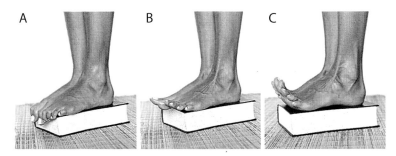

6 **Toe control:** Sit or lie with legs straight in front of you. Hold your feet at right angles to the floor and try to spread out your toes as far as you can. Then try to work each toe up and down individually. Repeat 10 times. (At first you will find it almost impossible to do this exercise, but in the beginning, try holding four toes and let the free one work individually.)

A   B   C

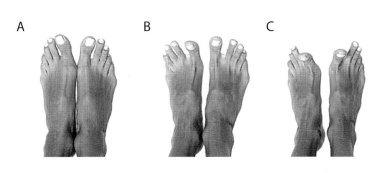

7 **Foot circles:** Sit or lie with legs stretched in front of you. Use one foot to make wide circles outward, arching the foot as you do it. Repeat 10 times. Then do 10 inward circles. Repeat with the other foot. This exercise improves the shape of the foot, and strengthens and trims down your ankles.

A   B   C

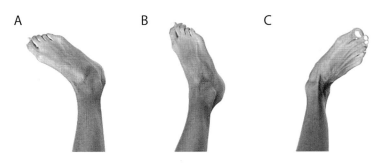

8 **Arch strengthener:** Using a foot roller on the floor, roll along the entire length of the foot. Roll backward and forward 10 times, concentrating on the arches. Repeat on other foot. This also relieves fatigue and cramping.

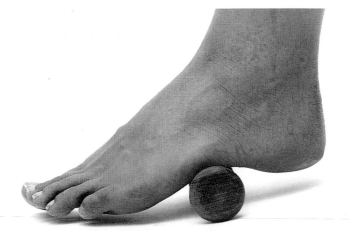

Massage therapies

A massage quickly revives tired feet. Use a refreshing cream or oil (with peppermint, for instance) and work your thumbs in a circular motion, starting at the ball of your foot, moving backward toward your heel. Return to the toes, massaging each individually. For more about massage techniques, *see* pages 122–123.

Wooden foot rollers, which come in all shapes and sizes, offer an easy alternative to massage. If you cannot find one, an old-fashioned rolling pin can be used at a pinch. Simply place the rolling pin on the floor and place your foot on it. Roll along the entire length of the foot, backward and forward, concentrating on the arches. Do this rolling 10 times, then swap to the other foot and repeat. This helps to strengthen your arches and to relieve fatigue and cramping.

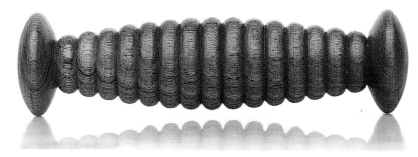

A wooden foot roller makes a useful substitute for a relaxing massage.

becomes sluggish and blocked due to stress, flows freely again.

As an alternative, walking barefoot on pebbles is also a good way to invigorate blocked energy.

Reflexology

An ancient technique practised for thousands of years, reflexology involves therapeutic massage of pressure points on the soles of the feet to stimulate major organs and aid in the excretion of toxins. There are reflex points on the

hands as well as the feet, so reflexologists can work on these too, although most of them prefer working on the feet because there are more reflex points there.

Reflexologists suggest that energy flows through our bodies in 10 zones. These run from the head down to the toes and the fingers, which are rich in nerve endings. The flow of energy – what the Chinese call *chi* – ends in many reflex points in the hands and feet.

Shiatsu

If you are stressed, a professional shiatsu massage will ease tension. It is an invigorating massage rather than a relaxing experience.

The Japanese interpretation of Chinese acupuncture, shiatsu (which means 'finger pressure') involves the exertion of firm pressure on various points of the body that relate to different organs and energy pathways. This addresses imbalances and ensures that the body's energy, which often

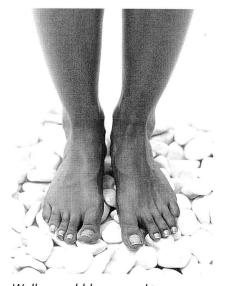 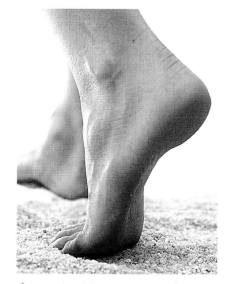

Walk on pebbles or sand to massage your feet and unblock energy pathways.

FOOT REFLEXOLOGY POINTS

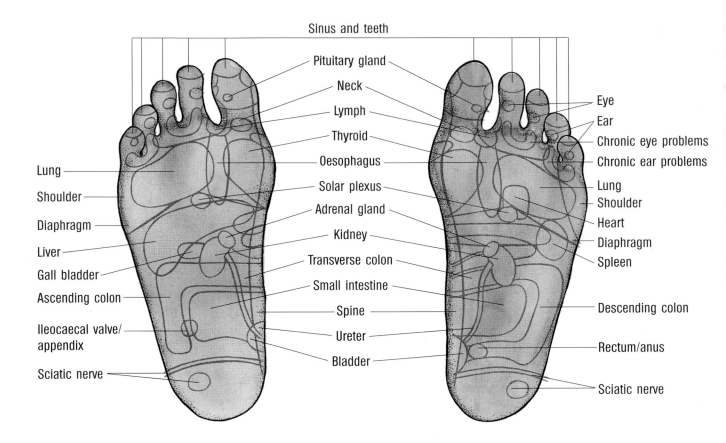

Sinus and teeth

Pituitary gland
Neck
Lymph
Thyroid
Oesophagus
Solar plexus
Adrenal gland
Kidney
Transverse colon
Small intestine
Spine
Ureter
Bladder

Lung
Shoulder
Diaphragm
Liver
Gall bladder
Ascending colon
Ileocaecal valve/
appendix
Sciatic nerve

Eye
Ear
Chronic eye problems
Chronic ear problems
Lung
Shoulder
Heart
Diaphragm
Spleen

Descending colon

Rectum/anus

Sciatic nerve

Different parts of the toes and feet relate to various organs or systems in the body. For example, the big toe corresponds to the head and the brain, the heel relates to the lower back, and the ball of the foot to the lungs.

If an area of the foot feels particularly tender, to a trained reflexologist this pain indicates tension or congestion in the related part of the body. The theory is that if there is an imbalance in the body, the energy becomes blocked at the reflex points, where toxins (uric crystals) will form.

A reflexologist can feel these blockages and will massage them to break down the crystals and restore the flow of energy. The massage may be gentle or deep depending on the degree of blockage. It will also stimulate the circulatory and lymphatic systems, and help to flush away any toxins.

Reflexology can help alleviate stress and anxiety, headaches, migraines, insomnia, asthma, eczema, premenstrual tension, digestive disorders, back pain and high blood pressure. (*See also pages 24–25 and page 104.*)

Reflexology treats the body and mind, so expect fairly detailed lifestyle questions at your first appointment. The therapist will normally start with a general foot massage, familiarizing herself with your feet and helping you relax, before going on to work on specific areas. It is not painful, although there may be some tenderness in places where there is congestion. During the treatment you may feel hot or cold as energy shifts around your body. You will probably feel tired, but relaxed, after the treatment.

DIY REFLEXOLOGY

Although not a substitute for professional treatment, gentle, generalized foot massage techniques are suitable for home use, too. Stretching and loosening the feet will improve local circulation and promote relaxation. Using steady, fairly firm pressure, you may locate tender spots on the feet. Treat these gently and do not press too hard or for too long as this can produce a strong reaction in the affected area of the body.

1 Massage each toe in turn using your thumb, then flex and extend gently. Twist foot sideways to stretch all the muscles.

2 Holding the top of the foot with one hand. Cup the heel in the other hand and use the top hand to flex and extend the foot to loosen the joints.

3 Ease out tension in the lateral arch by holding the foot with one hand on each side, and stretching across the top of the foot.

4 Knead and rub across the top and the sole of the foot, about 2.5cm (1in) away from the toes.

5 Apply gentle pressure to the solar plexus reflex – found between the big toe and the next toe, just below the large pad beneath the big toe. Pressing this point on both feet simultaneously is effective.

6 Hold the feet by resting your hands on top of them for a few minutes.

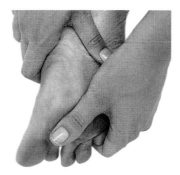

1 MASSAGE

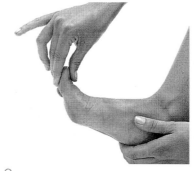

2 FLEX AND EXTEND

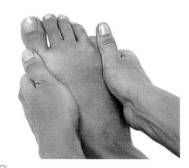

3 EASE TENSION

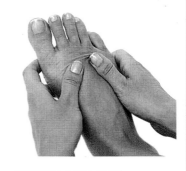

4 KNEAD AND RUB

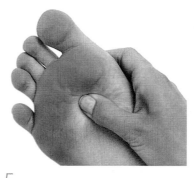

5 SOLAR PLEXUS POINT

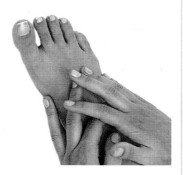

6 HOLD

USEFUL PRESSURE POINTS TO KNOW:

1 **Stimulate the brain:** press all over the pad of your big toe.

2 **Sinus headache:** squeeze the sides and back of each of your toes.

3 **Forehead headache** (probably been brought on by general tiredness): press just below the big toenail. Another point for general stress and headache relief is located four finger widths below the knee, outside the shinbone.

4 **Shoulder tension/pain:** pinch, press and gently hold the point between the bases of the fourth and fifth toes for a count of five.

5 **General stress relief:** the main pressure point is on the top of your foot where the big toe and second toe meet. Putting pressure on this point will also relieve headaches.

6 **Insomnia:** massage the point four finger-widths above the anklebone, on the inside of the leg, close to the shinbone.

7 **Indigestion, heartburn and nausea:** rub the spot situated between the second and third toes, where the bones meet on the top of your foot.

8 **Nausea:** thumb-walk over the entire area of the foot arch, which is linked to the abdomen. Concentrate on any tender areas, kneading them gently with your thumb. Then work the solar plexus area; this is just below the pads beneath the big and second toe. Try getting a partner to take both of your feet together and to press firmly on the solar plexus area as you inhale, and then release as you breathe out. Repeat this several times until the nausea is relieved.

9 **Neck strain:** walk your thumb up the outside edge of the underside of the big toe. Repeat on the same part of each toe on both feet. Then walk your thumb along the ridge immediately under the toes.

10 **Irritability:** firmly massage the solar plexus area (see point 8) on both feet at the same time. Then move your thumb down and 2.5cm (1in) across toward the baby toes to stimulate that area, which represents your liver.

Ageing feet

As you age, your feet develop more problems because the skin tends to become thin and lose its elasticity. Healing can take longer, and wear and tear to the joints over the years may cause some degree of arthritis (*see* page 21).

But painful and uncomfortable feet are not a natural part of growing old or something you simply have to 'put up with'. Much can be done to improve comfort, relieve pain and maintain mobility. Elderly people often need assistance with foot care, so a regular visit to a podiatrist is a good idea.

The older you get, the more you need a shoe that holds your foot firmly in place and gives you adequate support. Throw out those sloppy old favourites that may make you unstable when you walk. Instead, look for shoes with uppers of soft leather or a stretchy man-made fabric, which is also breathable. Avoid plastic easy-clean uppers that do not allow the foot to breathe and will not stretch to accommodate your own foot shape. Many shoes have cushioning or shock-absorbing soles to give you extra comfort when you walk.

Your shoes should be roomy enough, particularly if you intend to wear them every day. If you suffer with swollen feet, it is a good idea to put your shoes on as soon as you wake up, before your feet have had a chance to swell.

FOOT PACIFIERS FOR ACHING FEET

After a long day on your feet, there is nothing like a revitalizing footbath to ease uncomfortable aches and pains. Add six drops of aromatherapy peppermint oil to a bowl of hot (but not too hot) water. Swish it around and sit comfortably with both feet in the water. Relax or read a book while the peppermint oil soothes and tones. Pat your feet dry and gently massage in some relaxing oil. Geranium oil is good for general circulation problems; lemongrass oil helps improve energy, builds resistance to fatigue and is soothing for tired legs and venous (vein) conditions; peppermint oil is cooling and has anti-inflammatory properties; rosemary oil is useful for fluid retention; sage oil is an antiseptic, astringent stimulant that is ideal for fluid retention and general aches and pains; and lavender is particularly effective in helping to combat odorous feet.

Other good ideas for aching feet are:
- **Kick off your shoes and lift your feet onto a desk or table, or lie on your bed with your feet raised on two pillows.**
- **Wrap ice cubes in a flannel and rub it over your feet up to each ankle. Dry each foot and dab with witch-hazel.**
- **Rub your soles with cider vinegar or lemon juice.**
- **Soak your feet in a bowl of lukewarm water containing a spa solution or good old-fashioned Epsom salts. Apply a cooling foot lotion over your feet and legs, up to your knees.**

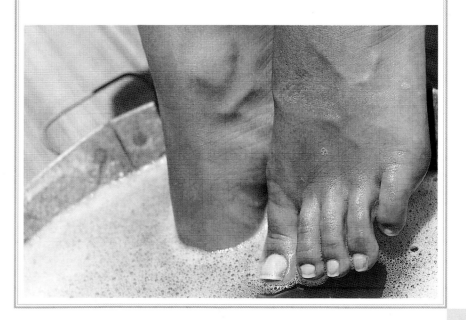

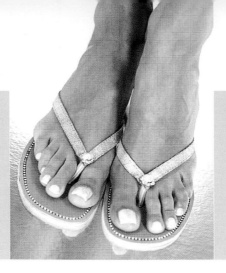

Pedicures: step by step

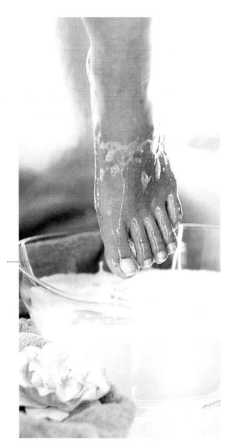

To perform a pedicure you will use all the tools required for a manicure (*see* pages 41–42) but will want to replace the finger bowl with a footbath. You will also need to add the following items to your kit:

- toenail nippers to allow you to achieve a precise trim
- foot file paddle to file away rough, callused skin
- antiseptic spray to sanitize your feet and prevent infection
- toe separators (moulded rubber devices) to prevent smudging while you apply polish.

Place a large folded terry towel on the floor in front of you and set the footbath on it once you have part-filled it with water. Add a few drops of liquid soap, essential oils or your favourite foot/bath salts to the water and allow them to disperse.

Place all your implements, files and supplies on a terry towel within easy reach. For any basic pedicure, you will be following the same type of procedures as with a manicure, although the files you use will be coarser because toenails are generally thicker than fingernails.

Above: Use as a footbath any container big enough to hold the foot. Right: Toe separators prevent polish from smudging.

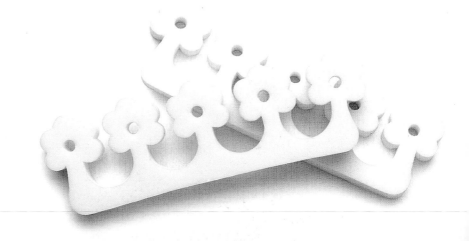

Pedicure kit essentials

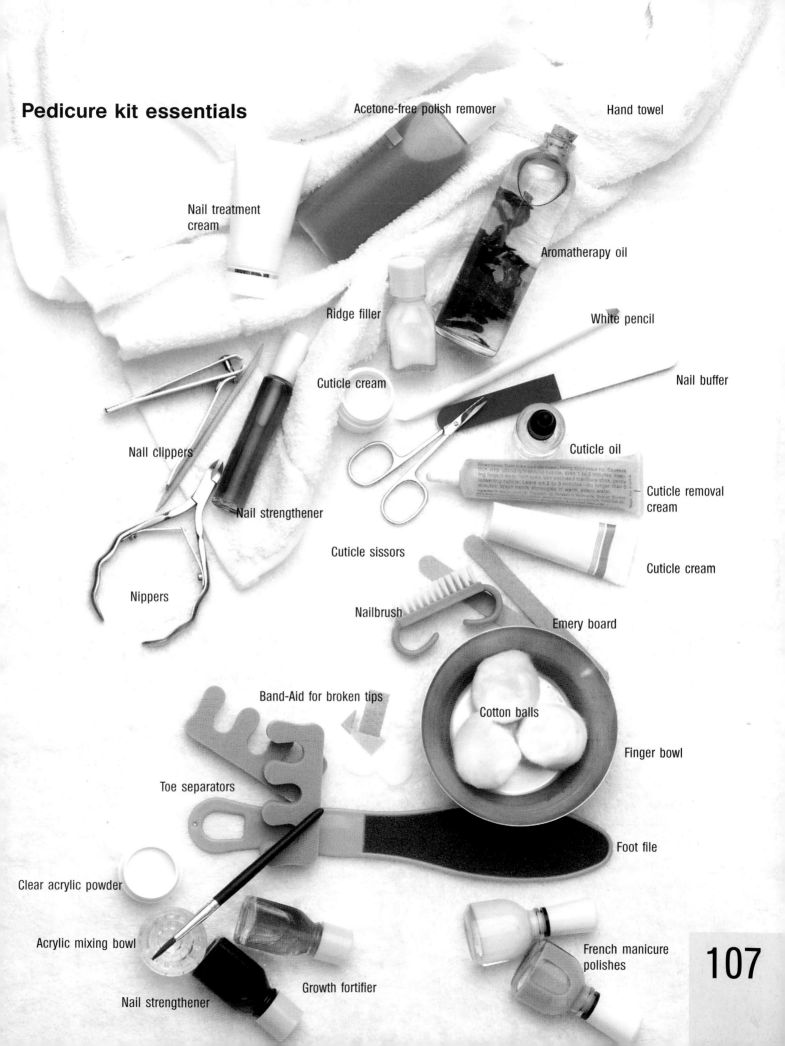

Acetone-free polish remover

Hand towel

Nail treatment cream

Aromatherapy oil

Ridge filler

White pencil

Cuticle cream

Nail buffer

Nail clippers

Cuticle oil

Nail strengthener

Cuticle removal cream

Cuticle sissors

Cuticle cream

Nippers

Nailbrush

Emery board

Band-Aid for broken tips

Cotton balls

Toe separators

Finger bowl

Foot file

Clear acrylic powder

Acrylic mixing bowl

French manicure polishes

Nail strengthener

Growth fortifier

Home pedicure

Are your heels dry and cracked and your toenails neglected? Remember that spending time caring for your feet should be an essential part of your beauty routine.

1 Remove old polish from the nails of both feet with nail varnish remover. Gently rub cuticle oil into the cuticles.

2 File toenails straight across, rounding slightly at the corners to conform to the shape of the toe. Use a fine file to smooth the underside of the corners and to bevel the free edge. Use the toenail nippers to remove the underside of the corners so they do not dig into your flesh to cause ingrown toenails. Buff nails to smooth out ridges and leave them shiny and healthy (great if you are not applying polish).

3 Apply cuticle softener and massage into the cuticle.

4 Use an orange stick or metal cuticle pusher to push back the transparent cuticle and to clean under the free edge. Never dig into the flesh, which may cause an infection. Do not use excessive pressure to push back your cuticles as this could result in damage to the matrix.

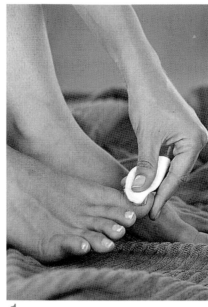
1 **REMOVE VARNISH**

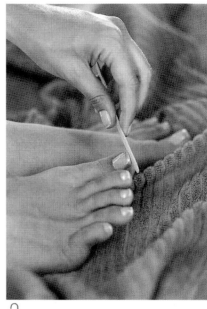
2 **FILE NAILS**

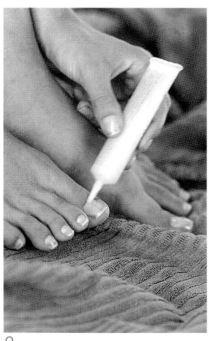
3 **APPLY CUTICLE SOFTENER**

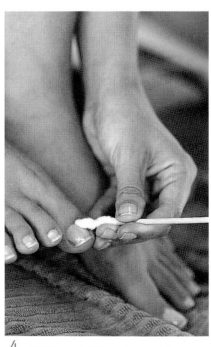
4 **PUSH BACK CUTICLES**

5   If you have loose cuticle skin or hangnails, remove this by nipping with the cuticle nippers, being very careful not to cut any live tissue.

6   Repeat steps 2–5 on the other foot.

7   If you have a build-up of callused skin, file it with a foot file paddle. Never use a corn or callus trimmer to cut or remove callused skin; it is too easy to remove healthy skin along with the callus. Never try to remove all of the callused skin in a single session. Depending on the depth of your callus, it can take several months or more for the healthy skin to show through.

8   Exfoliate the feet, including the soles, using dampened sea-salt or a suitable exfoliator to rub off rough skin patches and rev up your circulation.

9   Place feet into warm water in the footbath; flip on the massage button if your machine has one. Allow feet to soak for five minutes, adding either oils such as peppermint, or a specifically designed foot soak to soften and relax feet. Dry feet thoroughly.

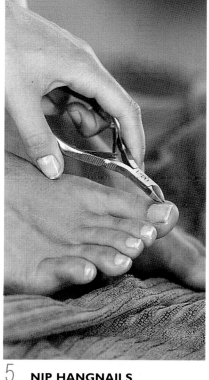

5 **NIP HANGNAILS**

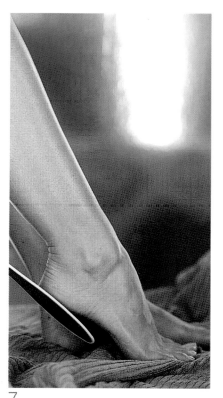

7 **FILE CALLUSES**

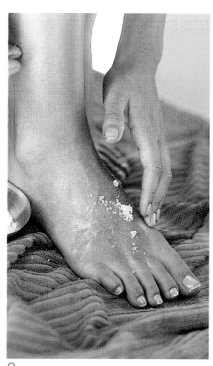

8 **EXFOLIATE**

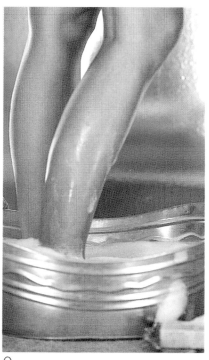

9 **SOAK**

10 Scrub your feet and toenails with the nailbrush, being sure to cleanse the side nail fold and under the free edge. Use a soft towel to dry your feet, legs and toes, not forgetting between the toes.

11 Massage both feet by applying lotion, cream or oil to the palms of your hands and then to your feet. Massage feet, lower legs and toes, then put both feet back into the footbath to remove all traces of oil or lotion. Wipe each toenail with a cottonwool or gauze pad saturated with remover or alcohol to ensure the nail plate is free of oils.

12 Apply a thin basecoat.

13 Apply two thin coats of colour and a thin topcoat for a long-lasting finish. Allow a minimum of one minute between coatings for each coat to dry. To prevent smudging, use toe separators. Leave in place until the enamel has dried completely.

14 Apply a spritz of refreshing mist, followed by moisturizer. Finally, empty the footbath and clean it, as well as all implements, with disinfecting solution. Make sure you dry them well before storing them in a sealed container.

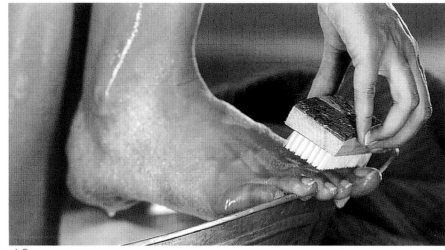
10 **SCRUB**

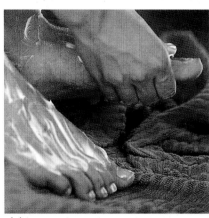
11 **MASSAGE**

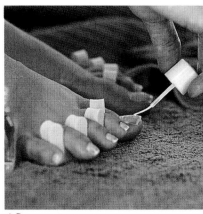
12 **APPLY BASECOAT**

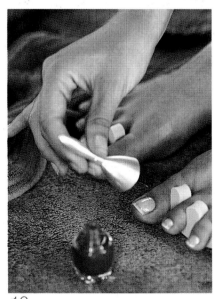
13 **APPLY VARNISH**

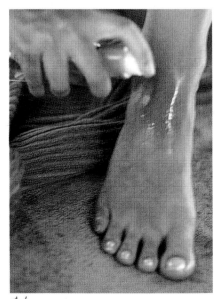
14 **SPRITZ WITH WATER**

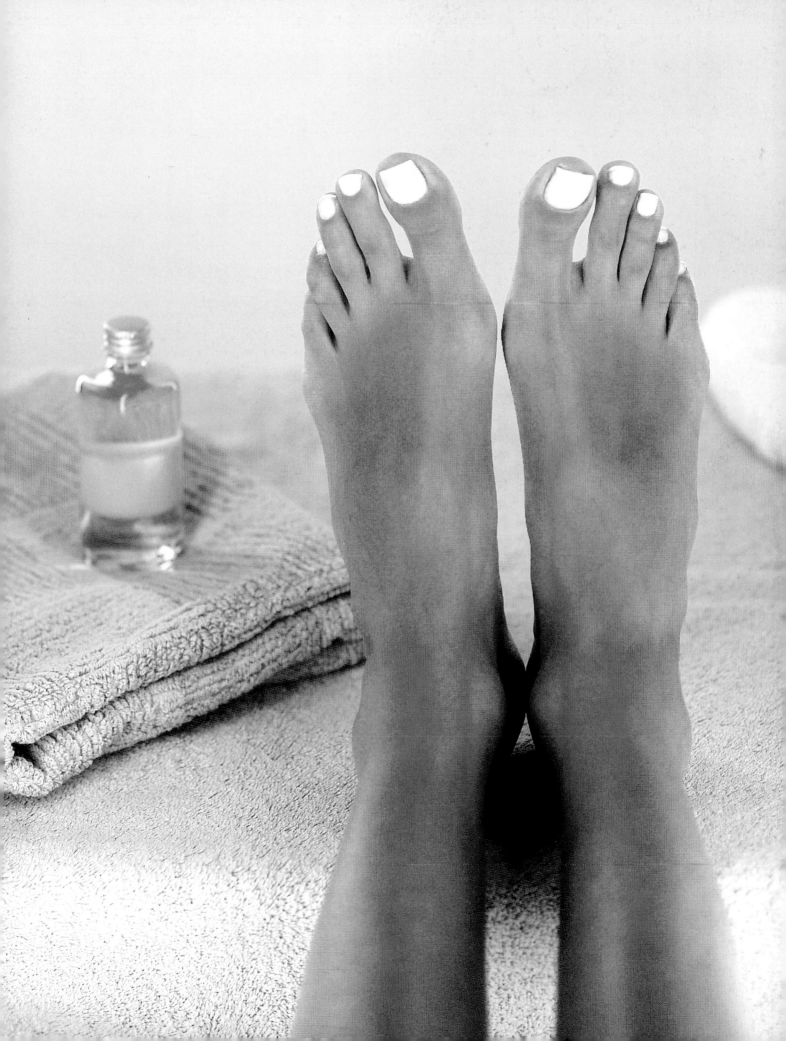

The salon pedicure

Feet are often neglected. Hidden away under layers of socks in winter and squashed into shoes all year round, they need special reviving care. For a special treat, nothing beats a salon pedicure.

1   Feet and legs are disinfected and dried, then the nails are trimmed so that they are even with the end of the toe.

2   Nails are filed straight across, rounding slightly at the corners to smooth jagged edges.

3   Cuticle softener is applied, and cuticles coaxed back with a specially designed hoof stick.

4   Dead skin and hangnails are clipped away with a pair of nippers.

5   Toenails are buffed with a buffer to remove ridges or any unevenness.

6   Nails are cleaned under the free edge with a cotton-wrapped orange stick or a special tool to remove any bits of cuticle and debris.

7   Feet are soaked in a vibrating footbath filled with water and a few drops of tea-tree oil, which has both antibacterial and antifungal properties. Smooth basalt pebbles are dropped into the footbath for a tactile experience.

8   Nails are scrubbed to remove any traces of cuticle cream or solvents.

9   A foot file/rasp is used on the ball and heel of the foot to remove dry skin and calluses. Some salons use an electric file to speed up this process.

10 Feet, ankles and calves are massaged with aloe vera gel.

11 Hot basalt and cool marble stones are used to alternate temperatures and enhance the sensory experience of a stone massage.

12 The reflexology points on the soles of the feet are massaged using the cool and gentle pressure of the marble stones.

13 Pebbles are placed between the toes to stretch them and help alleviate stiffness.

14 Disposable toe separators are placed between the toes, traces of lotion removed and basecoat applied, then two layers of colour and topcoat. Finally, feet are rested on the pebbles until the varnish dries.

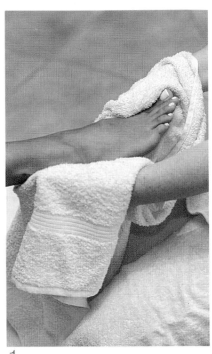

1   **DISINFECT, TRIM AND DRY**

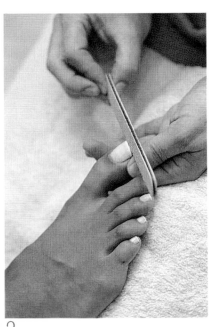

2   **FILE**

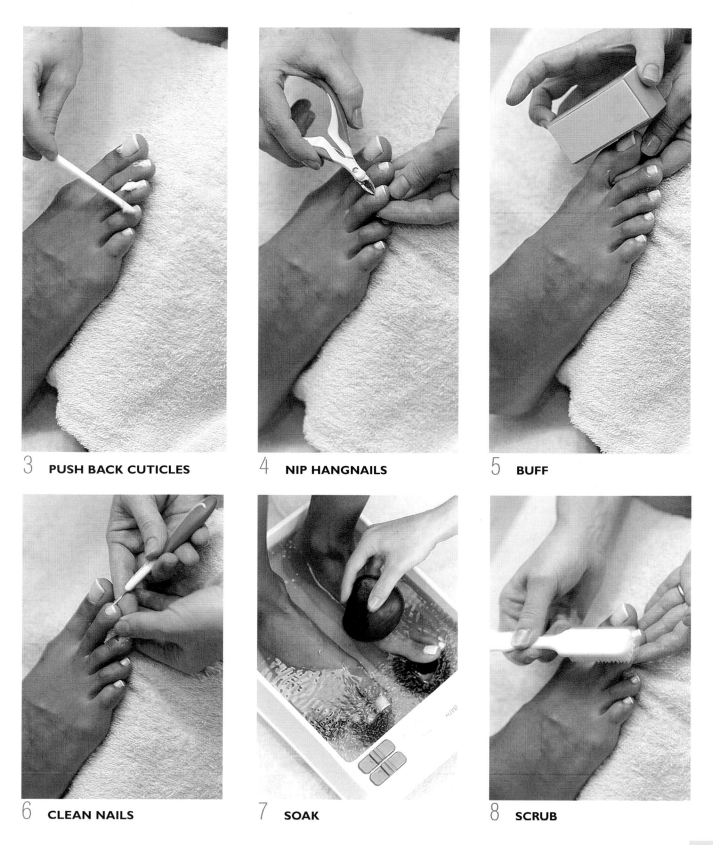

3 PUSH BACK CUTICLES

4 NIP HANGNAILS

5 BUFF

6 CLEAN NAILS

7 SOAK

8 SCRUB

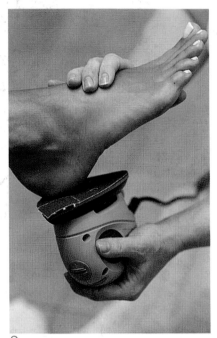

9 **REMOVE CALLUSES**

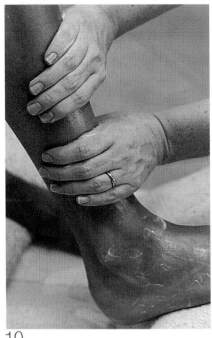

10 **MASSAGE**

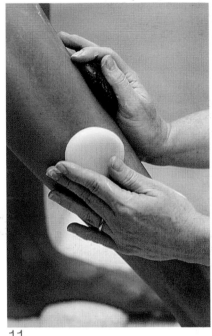

11 **HOT/COLD PEBBLES**

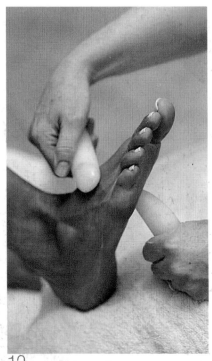

12 **REFLEXOLOGY**

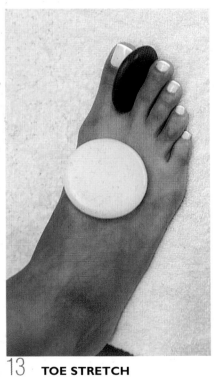

13 **TOE STRETCH**

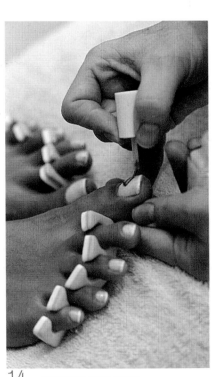

14 **APPLY VARNISH**

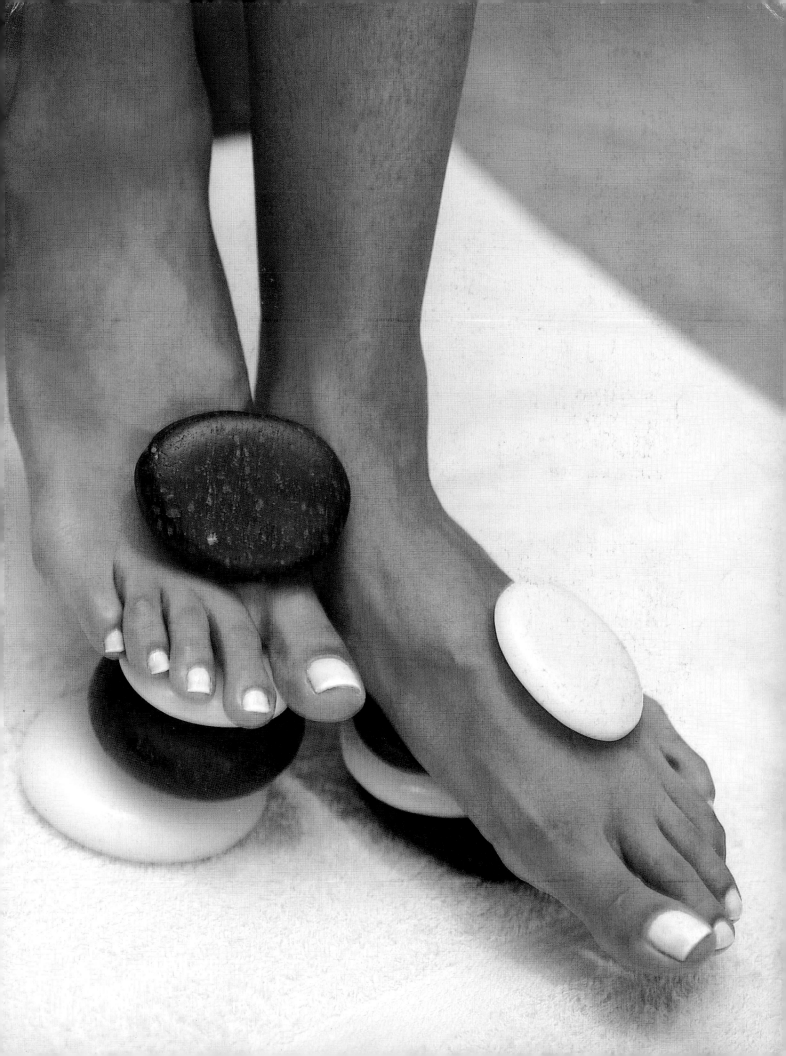

The French pedicure

If your toenails are not your best feature, opt for clear, pearlized or pale-coloured nail varnish so as not to draw too much attention to them. A French pedicure is a neutral option that makes almost any foot look good.

1 Follow the basic steps for a pedicure until you have applied basecoat (*see* pages 108–110).

2 Apply white polish to the nail tip by starting at one side and sweeping across the nail in a single, steady movement. Keep the strip as narrow as possible. Repeat for all the nails. If you find this too difficult to achieve neatly, opt for some self-adhesive French manicure guides mentioned on page 56.

3 Apply sheer pink, natural or peach polish over the entire nail, painting a strip of colour down the centre of the nail, then overlapping with a strip on either side, but avoiding the cuticles. Leave to dry thoroughly before applying a second coat.

4 Apply a clear topcoat to seal in colour. Leave to dry for as long as possible before putting on your shoes – at least an hour, as socks or tights can leave unsightly imprints if you rush the drying stage.

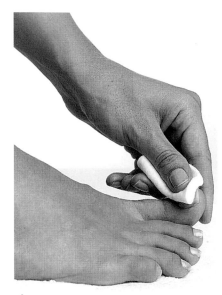

1 **REMOVE OLD POLISH**

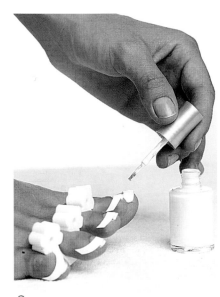

2 **PAINT TIPS WHITE**

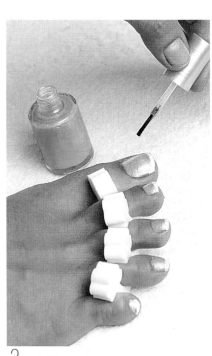

3 **APPLY SHEER VARNISH**

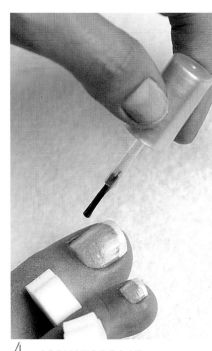

4 **APPLY TOPCOAT**

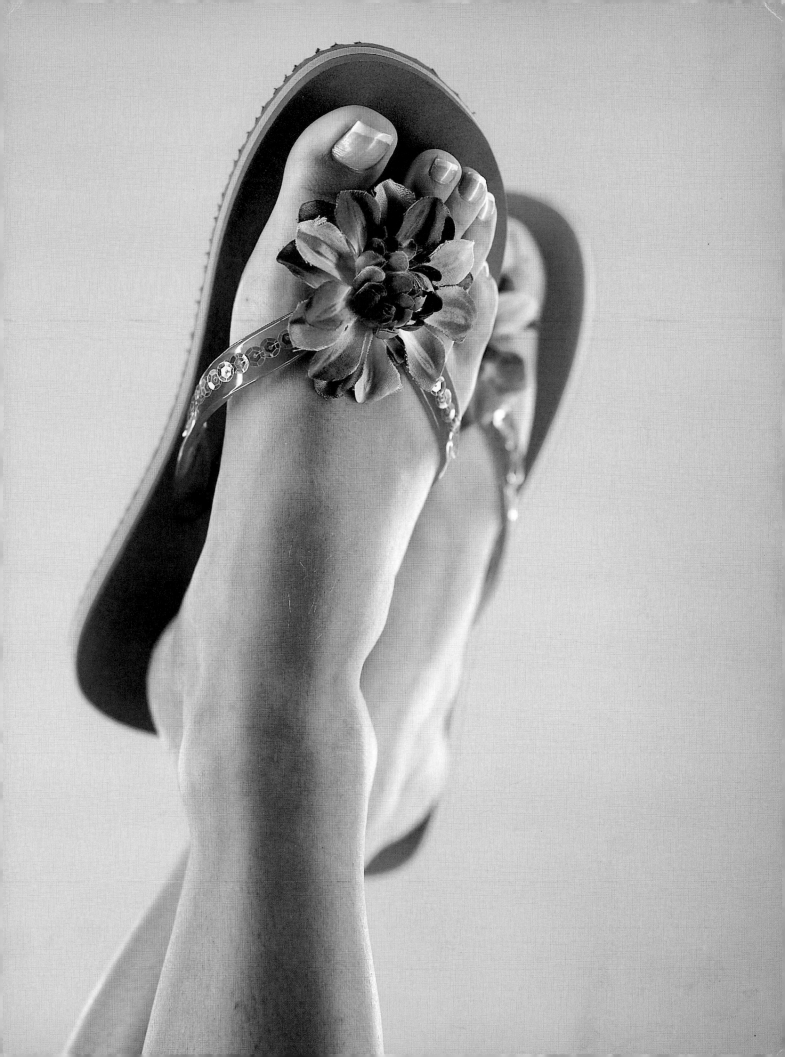

Fashion feet

Nail colour is an instant accessory. Fun and cheap, it will really make your feet pretty for a night on the town.

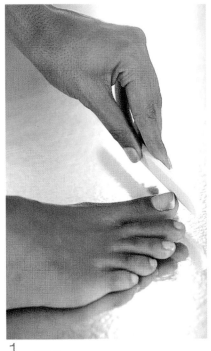

1 **FILE**

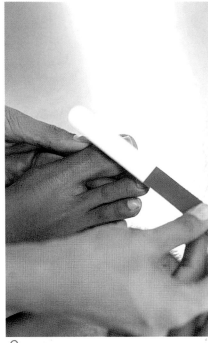

2 **BUFF**

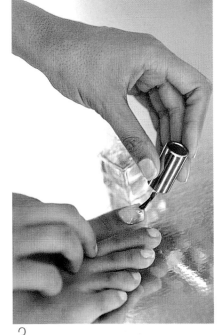

3 **APPLY BASECOAT**

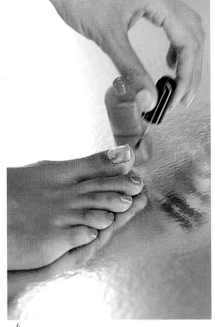

4 **APPLY COLOUR**

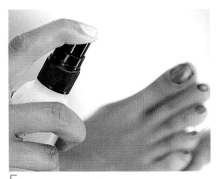

5 **USE INSTANT NAIL DRY**

1 File the nails straight across with an emery board. Smooth the edges with the finer side. Moisturize cuticles and gently push back with an orange stick tipped with cotton wool.

2 Buff out any ridges or uneven-ness with a buffer.

3 Remove traces of lotion or cuticle softener and apply one coat of ridge-filler or the basecoat of your choice.

4 Apply two coats of your favourite high-fashion varnish shade, or see 'fashion tips' (right) for other fun ideas. Finally, apply a topcoat for endurance.

5 Spray with instant nail dry or allow to dry naturally for a longer-lasting pedicure.

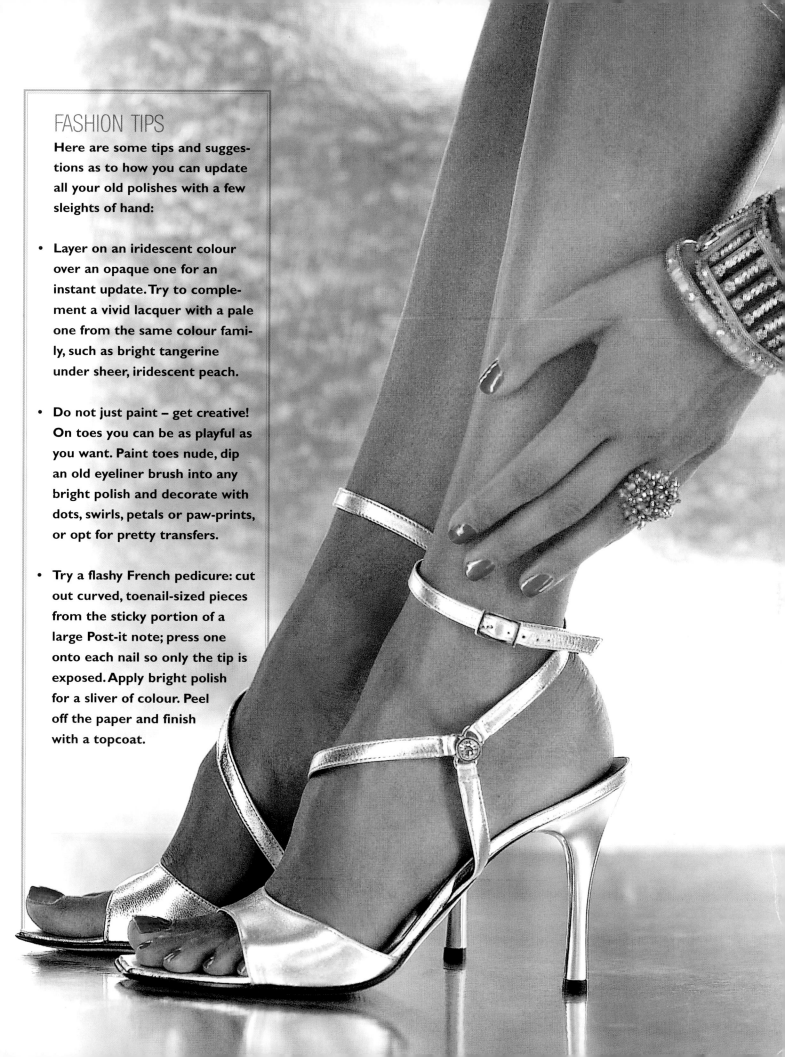

FASHION TIPS

Here are some tips and suggestions as to how you can update all your old polishes with a few sleights of hand:

- Layer on an iridescent colour over an opaque one for an instant update. Try to complement a vivid lacquer with a pale one from the same colour family, such as bright tangerine under sheer, iridescent peach.

- Do not just paint – get creative! On toes you can be as playful as you want. Paint toes nude, dip an old eyeliner brush into any bright polish and decorate with dots, swirls, petals or paw-prints, or opt for pretty transfers.

- Try a flashy French pedicure: cut out curved, toenail-sized pieces from the sticky portion of a large Post-it note; press one onto each nail so only the tip is exposed. Apply bright polish for a sliver of colour. Peel off the paper and finish with a topcoat.

Spa treat with floral soak and foot mask

Aromatherapy massage, body wraps and masks come in a variety of guises. From the exotic experience of a rose-oil wrap to the deep-cleansing properties of a kaolin or mud pack, there are many alternatives to play with, so get creative and create your own spa experience.

1 Treat feet to a restorative foot-bath. Fill a bowl with warm water, throw in fresh flowers or rose petals, light some candles, put on some meditative music and sit back and relax.

2 Soak your feet in hot water for 10 to 15 minutes, dropping in a few drops of peppermint oil to refresh or a few drops of lavender oil to relax.

3 Vaporizing essential oils in a burner will provide the room with a continuous fragrance. Try relaxing rose geranium or lavender, or invigorating peppermint or grapefruit.

4 Body brushing improves your circulation and helps to eliminate toxins from the body by boosting the lymphatic system. The exfoliating effect sloughs away dead skin cells. Brush in one direction from the soles of your feet up along your legs using gentle but firm pressure.

5 A salt scrub gives instant relief and ongoing therapy for troublesome joints, overworked muscles and fluid retention. By improving circulation it also ensures even skin tone. Perk up circulation and buff your skin with a commercial scrub or this mixture: 30 drops of lavender aromatherapy oil, 125ml carrier oil, 50g coarse sea salt. Dampen feet and exfoliate them (or the whole body if you like), working upward from the toes. Shower or rinse off with warm water and pat dry.

6 Eliminate any unsightly dark hairs on your toes with bleach or pre-waxed strips.

7 Treat tired feet to an indulgent mudpack or mask. Place feet on clingfilm, then brush on the mask. Use a commercial product or this mixture: 150g Fuller's earth, 200ml water, 2 drops vetiver, 2 drops frankincense, 4 drops lavender oil, a tablespoon honey.

8 Wrap feet in clingfilm and leave for 15 minutes. Rinse with warm water and pat dry.

9 Massage with cool quartz crystals. Place a large crystal under your foot and apply gentle pressure to the solar plexus reflex point, rolling the arch of your foot backward and forward over the crystal.

10 Slough off rough or callused skin with a foot file.

11 Apply a generous layer of lavender-based foot cream to soothe aches and pains.

12 Massage cream thoroughly all over your toes and toenails using thumb and index fingers. With the sole facing downward, pinch the web between toes to drain your feet. Use the thumb on the upperside and your middle three fingers on the sole to give the soles a final rub.

Left: Lavender aromatherapy oil adds to the relaxing experience.

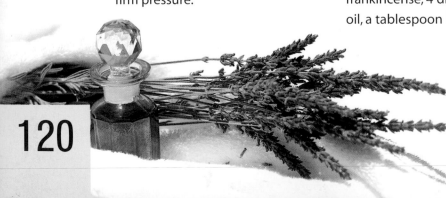

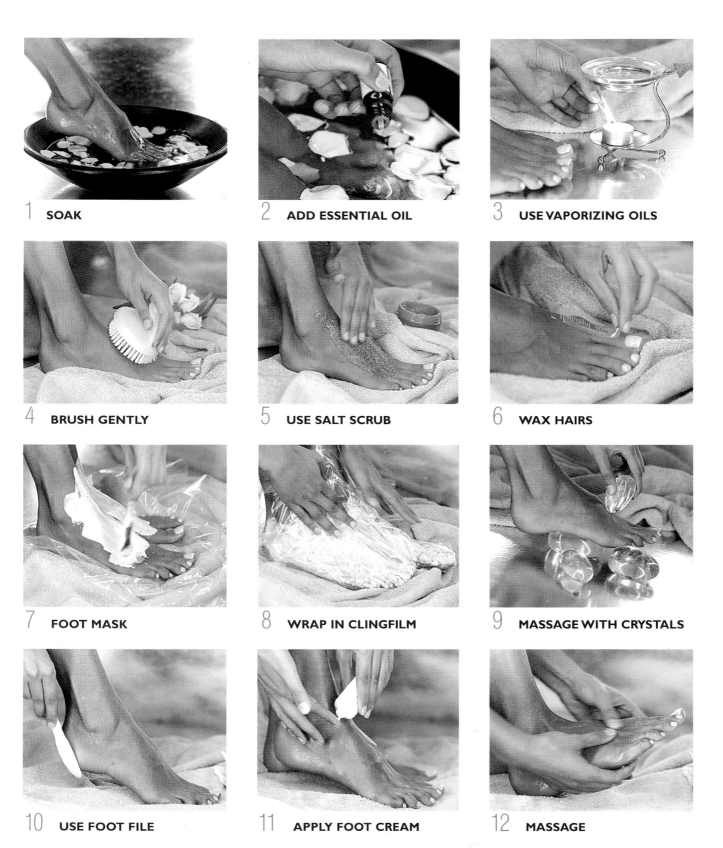

1 SOAK

2 ADD ESSENTIAL OIL

3 USE VAPORIZING OILS

4 BRUSH GENTLY

5 USE SALT SCRUB

6 WAX HAIRS

7 FOOT MASK

8 WRAP IN CLINGFILM

9 MASSAGE WITH CRYSTALS

10 USE FOOT FILE

11 APPLY FOOT CREAM

12 MASSAGE

Massage techniques

A foot massage can be performed at any time or as part of your home pedicure. If you are using massage oil or lotion, a towel will come in handy to protect the floor and furniture. Follow these steps for a simple DIY massage.

1 Rub oiled or creamed hands vigorously to warm them before starting your massage.

2 Gentle stroking stimulates the circulation and boosts lymphatic drainage. Starting on the top of the foot, begin a slow, firm stroking motion with your hands. Begin at the tips of the toes and slide all the way to the ankle, then retrace your steps to the toes with a lighter stroke. Repeat five times.

3 Next, stroke the top of the foot with your thumbs, starting at the base of the toes and moving over top of instep while fingers move from the ball of the foot, over the arch, to the heel and back again. Use long firm strokes, slightly pressing with your thumbs as you go. Repeat five times.

4 Starting with the big toe, gently stroke each toe using an upward movement, sliding your fingers to the top and back to the base.

5 Hold the foot beneath the ankle, cupping the heel. Holding the toe with your thumb on top and index finger beneath and starting at the base of the toe, slowly and firmly pull or lift the toe, sliding your fingers to the top and back to the base. Repeat with each toe, gently squeezing and rolling the toe between your thumb and index fingers while working your way to the tip and back to the base.

6 Hold foot behind the ankle, cupping under the heel. Using the heel of your other hand, push hard as you slide along the arch from the ball of the foot toward the heel and back again. This releases tension in the inner and outer arches. Repeat a few times. Slightly firmer pressure is preferable here.

7 Hold the foot behind the ankle, cupping it to brace the foot and leg. Grasp the ball of the foot with one hand and turn the foot slowly at the ankle a few times in each direction. Press gently on the solar plexus pressure point (between the big toe and the next toe, just below the large pad beneath the big toe).

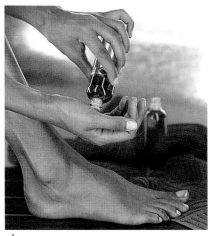

1 **OIL HANDS**

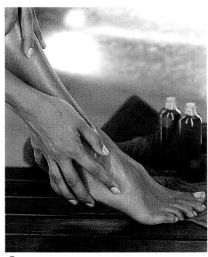

2 **STROKE TOP OF FOOT**

Gently press into this point and repeat a few times, moving down toward the heel and back again.

8 Repeat step 1 to complete the foot massage. Then repeat all steps on other foot.

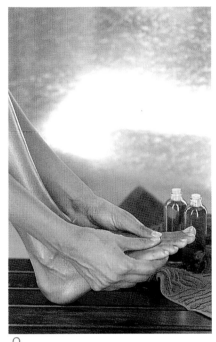

3   **STROKE WITH THUMBS**

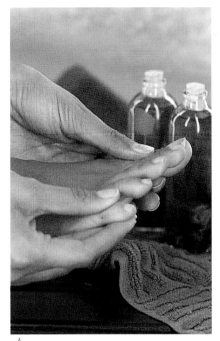

4   **STROKE TOES**

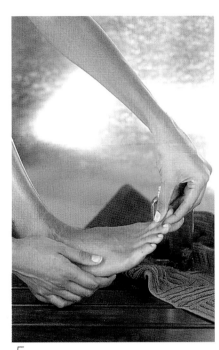

5   **PULL TOES**

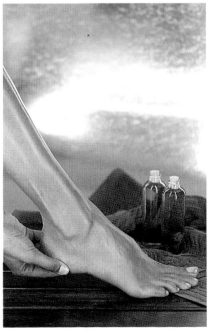

6   **MASSAGE ARCH TO HEEL**

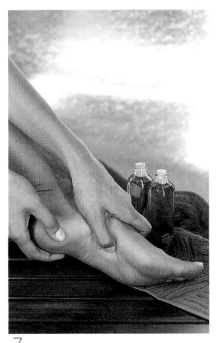

7   **APPLY PRESSURE**

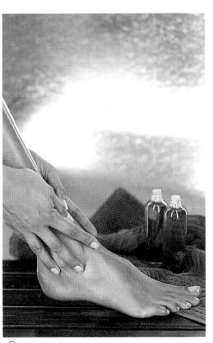

8   **STROKE**

Foot reflexology

Reflexology has been used to treat a number of common ailments, including back pain, digestive problems, migraine, menstrual problems, sinus problems and general stress and tension. Apart from helping to reduce pain, it is of considerable benefit in stress-related ailments. It is useful as a diagnostic aid, as tender reflex points can help locate areas of dysfunction. Although no substitute for a professional treatment, gentle, generalized foot massage techniques suitable for home use help to maintain good health. Arrange for your partner to be warm and comfortable, sitting with feet raised, ideally almost as high as your shoulders so that your arms will not tire.

1 Use your left hand as a support for the right foot, your right hand for the left foot. Cup the heel of the foot firmly so it rests in your hand, curving your fingers around the outside of the heel. Grasp the top of the foot near the base of the toes, thumb underneath and fingers on top. Use the top hand to flex and extend the foot to loosen up the joints.

2 Flex the foot, gently easing the heel toward you so that the Achilles tendon is stretched. Repeat a few times on each foot.

3 Position your hands so the base of each palm lies above the side of the heel, behind the anklebone. Cup your hands over the ankle joint.

4 Move your hands quickly back and forth in opposite directions to each other, shaking the foot from side to side until the foot feels relaxed.

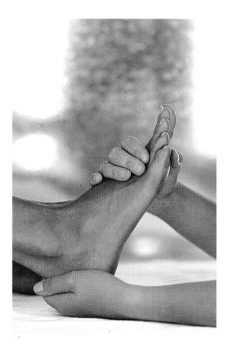

1 CUP HEEL

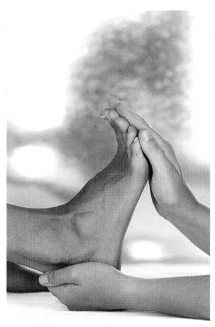

2 STRETCH

5 Hold the foot from the inside using both hands, fingers on top, thumbs on the sole. The hand closest to the toes will twist and work up and down while the other hand remains still. Work in small stages along the length of the foot.

6 Grasp the foot in both hands, with your hands clasped one on top of each other, and

wring gently (as you would a wet towel), hands twisting in opposite directions. Move your hands gradually up the foot, wringing the entire length as you go.

7 Massage each toe in turn, beginning with the big toe. Hold the base of the toe close to the base joint, with your thumb below and your index

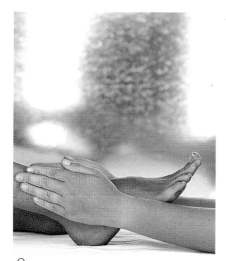

3   **CUP ANKLE**

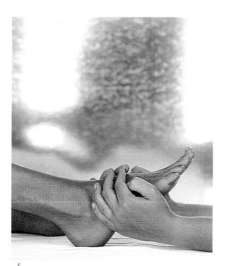

4   **SHAKE, SIDE TO SIDE**

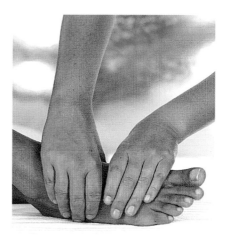

5   **HOLD AND TWIST**

and third finger on top. Gently lift the toe in its joint, rotating clockwise then anti-clockwise a few times.

8   Place the tips of your thumbs on the solar plexus reflex; press and release a few times. This point, a collection of nerve fibres that controls the digestive organs, is located between the big toe and the next toe. Note that pressing on both feet at the same time is more effective.

9   Flex the toes backward while supporting the heel, then rotate the foot in a circle, first clockwise a few times, then anti-clockwise. To finish, hold the feet by resting the hands gently on top of them for a few moments.

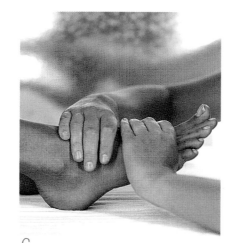

6   **WRING GENTLY**

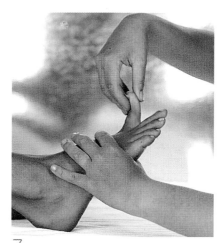

7   **MASSAGE TOES**

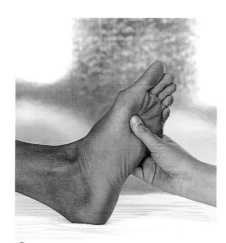

8   **PRESS REFLEX POINT**

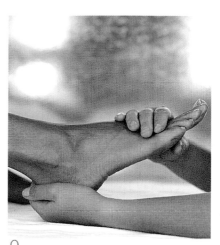

9   **HOLD FEET**

Glossary

Acetone: chemical in nail-varnish remover

Age spots: harmless dark brown skin patches; also known as liver spots

Blister: accumulation of blood or fluid between outer and inner skin layers; usually caused by friction

Buffer: padded implement to stimulate blood flow to nail bed to provide shine

Bunion: tender bump at the joint nearest the big toe

Bursa: fluid-filled sac in areas of pressure, e.g. joints

Bursitis: inflammation and swelling of the bursae

Callus: thickened patch of skin subjected to friction; also called keratoma

Carpal Tunnel Syndrome: pressure on median nerve of wrist causing numbness, pain, tingling fingers

Chi: Chinese concept of energy flow

Chilblains: itching sores or redness on hands and feet caused by exposure to cold

Collagen: fibre in dermis that gives skin its structure

Cuticle: thin tissue surrounding base of nail

Dermatitis: general term for skin inflammation with redness, pain, or itching

Dermis: inner layer of skin, located beneath epidermis

Elastin: elastic fibres that give skin its flexibility

Epicondylitis: pain and swelling of muscles and tendons around elbow; also called tennis elbow

Epidermis: outer layer of skin, over the dermis

Exfoliator: substance that sloughs off dead skin cells

Formaldehyde: preservative in nail hardeners/polish

Free edge: part of nail that extends over the fingertip

Furrow: nail corrugation (lengthwise or across)

Gout: metabolic disease associated with uric acid build-up in the blood and uric acid salts around joints

Hangnail: loose skin near cuticle or sides of the nail

Haematoma: bruising

Henna: vegetable tannin that stains skin/nails for decoration

Hoof stick: stick with a rubber tip (shaped like a hoof) used to push back cuticles

Hypertrophy: *see* onychauxis

Keratin: tough protein making up hair and nails

Keratoma: *see* callus

Koilonychia: spoon nails

Leuconychia: whitish nail discoloration (white spots)

Lunula: whitish half-moon at base of the nail

Macronychia: excessively large nails

Matrix: nail root where nail keratin is produced

Melanin: pigment that gives skin its colour and protects against UV rays

Melanonychia: darkening of finger- or toenails

Nail bed: finger tissue beneath nail plate

Nail folds: folds of skin at the nail base and sides that frame and support the nail

Nail fortifier: usually clear varnish containing calcium or growth formula

Nail plate: what most people call the nail

Nail sculpturing: technique using a product to build realistic artificial nails

Nail wrap: nail-sized pieces of cloth/paper bonded to the nail plate

Nipper: hangnail trimmer

Occupational Overuse Syndrome: term for a range of conditions characterized by discomfort/pain in muscles, tendons, and aggravated by repetitive movements

Onychatrophia: wasting away of the nail plate

Onychauxis: overgrowth/over-thickening/curving of nail; also called hypertrophy

Onychocryptosis: ingrown toenails

Onychogryposis: thickened, claw-like nails

Onychophagia: nail biting

Onychorrhexis: abnormally brittle nails

Orange stick: stick, made from orange tree wood, used to push back cuticles

Osteoarthritis: age-related degenerative condition attacking cartilage around weight-bearing joints

Paronychia: bacterial infection of the nail fold

Pseudomonas: bacterial infection between nail plate and nail bed

Psoriasis: chronic skin condition; red, thickened areas covered by silvery scales

Pterygium: inward advance of skin over the nail plate

Rheumatoid arthritis: chronic inflammatory disease in which cartilage of joints erodes, causing them to calcify and become immovable

Ridge filler: basecoat containing silk, talc or other particles to fill in depressions or ridges

Shiatsu: Japanese massage; means 'finger pressure'

Spoon nails: *see* koilonychia

Stratum corneum: outermost layer of the epidermis

Sun protection factor (SPF): indicator of how long you can be exposed to the sun before you burn, compared to using no sunscreen

Sunscreen: oil, lotion or cream containing compounds to filter out UV rays

UVA rays: sun rays that cause skin cancer and collagen breakdown

UVB rays: sun rays that cause tanning, burning and skin cancer

Warts: Skin growths caused by human papillomavirus infection in top skin layer/mucous membranes

Further reading and recommended websites

Ancient and Healing Art of Aromatherapy, The. Hill, Clare. London: Hamlyn (1997)

Beauty Wisdom. Vyas, Bharti and Haggard, Claire. London: Harper Collins (1998)

Body Shop Book, The. London: Little Brown & Co. (1994)

Book of Palmistry, The. Gettings, Fred. London: Hamlyn (1974)

Carpal Tunnel Syndrome. Montgomery, Kate. San Diego: Sports Touch Publishing (1994)

Complete Illustrated Guide to Reflexology. Dougans, Inge. London: Harper Collins (2001)

Consumer's Dictionary of Cosmetic Ingredients. Winter, R. New York: Three Rivers Press (1999)

Face of the Century, The – 100 Years of Makeup and Style. De Castelbajac, Kate.

Guide to Natural Therapies, The. Evans, Mark. London: Lorenz Books (1996)

Hands & Feet. Morley, C and Wilde, L. London: MQ Publications (2000)

Hands of Light. Brennan, Barbara Ann. New York: Bantam (1998) Harrold, Fiona. Headline (1994)

Healthy Feet. Russel, Lewis. London: Vintage/Edbury House (1998)

Holistix. Chaplin, Carole. London: Sidgewick & Jackson (1990)

Instant Nailcare. Norton, Sally. London: Anness Publishing (2000)

K.I.S.S. Guide to Beauty. Pedersen, Stephanie. London: Dorling Kindersley (2001)

Milady's Art & Science of Nail Technology. New York: Milady Publishing (1995)

Milady's Standard Textbook of Cosmetology. New York: Milady Publishing (1995)

Natural Hand Care. Pasekoff Weinberg, N. Vermont: Storey Books (1998)

Natural History of the Senses, A. Ackerman, Diane. New York: Random House (1990)

Runner's Repair Manual, The. Weisenfeld, M. and Burr, B. New York: St Martin's Press (1985)

Science of Beauty Therapy, The. Bennett, R. London: Hodder & Stoughton (1995)

Skin Source Book, The. Boyd, Alan S. Los Angeles: Lowell House (1998)

Touch for Health. Thie, Johan. California: TH Enterprises (1973).

Vital Oils. Earle, Liz. Ebury Press (1991)

www.feetforlife.org
a valuable guide to health, including advice on shoes, foot problems and how to maintain healthy feet and toenails

www.international-foot-and-shoe.com.au
all about keeping feet healthy and beautiful

www.waningmoon.com
a Gothic site that includes useful information on how to remove nail varnish stains, and details on acrylic nails. It also has useful information on nail care for men

www.stepwise-uk.com
a site that shows you how to maintain healthy toenails and feet

www.hooked-on-nails.com
learn about nail growth, nail health, nail care, and types of manicures and pedicures, as well as nail maintenance

www.anatomical.com
wealth of information about muscles and how they work, as well as a ready reference for anything anatomical; great resource for medical charts, diagrams and working models

www.fitnesszone.co.za
this is an excellent general fitness site that also has tons of step-by-step exercises for suitable for everyone, whatever your level of fitness

www.goodfeet.com
a great site that helps you to locate arch supports and orthoses, as well as cushion and comfort shoes

www.dreamyfeet.co.uk/
good source for products and information relating to foot pain

www.sallyhansen.com
lots of tips and pointers on nail colour and treatments, artificial nails, as well as hand and foot care

www.24dr.com/reference/library/skin/nails/footcare.htm
this easy-to-use diagnostic site has an excellent reference library; simply click on your symptoms to find out what the problem is and what to do about it

www.footcaredirect.com/
useful information on anything to do with the study and treatment of foot, ankle and heel conditions

www.womenfitness.net/beauty/handfeet/dodont.htm
valuable tips on hand and nail care, highlighting useful do's and don'ts

www.cir-safety.org
if you are concerned about the ingredients in nail products and treatments, this is the site for you; here you will find lists of cosmetic ingredients, as well as advice on possible allergic reactions or signs of poisoning

127

Index